SELF-ASSESSMENT PICTURE TESTS IN
VETERINARY MEDICINE

Clinical Anatomy

J. S. Boyd
BVMS PhD MRCVS
Professor in Veterinary Anatomy
The University of Glasgow
Veterinary School
Bearsden, Glasgow

M Mosby-Wolfe

London Baltimore Bogotá Boston Buenos Aires Caracas Carlsbad, CA Chicago Madrid Mexico City
Milan Naples, FL New York Philadelphia St. Louis Sydney Tokyo Toronto Wiesbaden

Project Manager:	Alison Taylor
Designer:	Judith Gauge
Cover Design:	Paul Phillips
Production:	Joe Lynch
Index:	Angela Cottingham
Publisher:	Jane Hunter

Contents

Acknowledgements

I should like to thank my co-workers from the *Color Atlas of Clinical Anatomy of the Dog and Cat* (published by Mosby-Wolfe, 1991) for use of illustrations from the book. I also wish to acknowledge my colleagues in the Department of Veterinary Anatomy at Glasgow University Veterinary School, especially Dr MD Purton and Dr ME Pirie for contributing a number of the photographs for this book.

Gross Anatomy

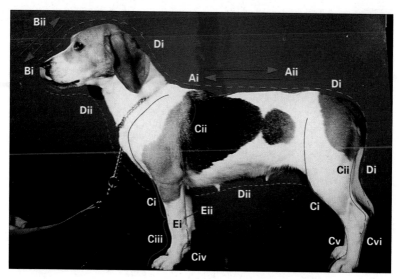

▲ 1.

(a) Give the correct directional anatomical terms indicated by the arrows **Ai** and **Aii**. Arrow **Ai** is pointing in what direction? Arrow **Aii** is pointing in what direction?

(b) Can the identical directional terms used in (a) be applied to describe the arrows marked **Bi** and **Bii**? Explain your answer giving names.

(c) Can the identical directional terms used in (a) be applied to describe the lines marked **Ci** and **Cii**; **Ciii** and **Civ**, **Cv** and **Cvi**? Explain your answer giving names.

(d) How would you describe the topographical anatomical term for the body region marked **Di** and **Dii**?

(e) What topographical term would you apply to describe the surface of the leg marked **Ei** to differentiate it from the surface of the opposite limb marked **Eii**?

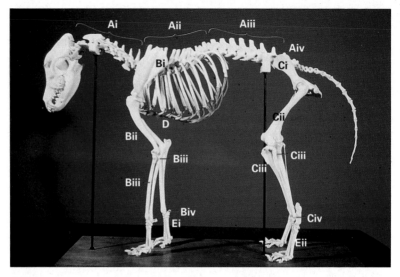

▲ 2.

(a) Identify and name the groups of bones marked **Ai**, **Aii**, **Aiii** and **Aiv** and give the normal number found in each group in this species.

(b) Identify and name the bones marked **Bi**, **Bii**, **Biii** and **Biv**.

(c) Identify and name the bones marked **Ci**, **Cii**, **Ciii** and **Civ**.

(d) Identify and name the bony structure marked **D** and state its normal components.

(e) Identify and name the group of bones marked **Ei** and **Eii** and state how many of each are normally found in the dog.

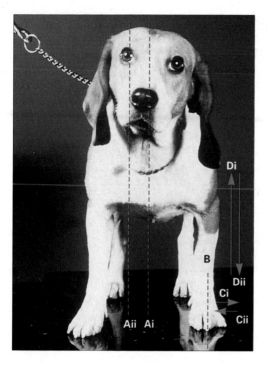

▲ 3.

(a) How would you describe in anatomical terms the plane of a section if it was made through the body along the line **Ai**? Could the same term be applied to a section along the line **Aii**? Explain your answer giving names.

(b) How would you describe in anatomical terms the plane of a section if it was made along line **B**?

(c) What directional anatomical terms could you apply to the directions indicated by the arrows **Ci** and **Cii**?

(d) What directional anatomical terms could you apply to the directions indicated by the arrows **Di** and **Dii**?

(e) How would you describe the aspect of the dog which you are looking at in this photograph? What would be the term you would use to describe the aspect of the dog that would be facing you if the dog was placed in the opposite direction?

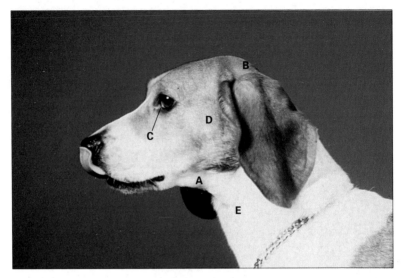

▲ **4.**

(a) Identify and name which semirigid structure could be palpated at **A**.

(b) Identify and name the bony protuberance which could be palpated subcutaneously at **B**. To which bone of the skull does it belong?

(c) Identify and name any orifice that you know of which could be found opening at the precise point **C**. What would be the function of this orifice and what might flow through it?

(d) What muscular structure would lie deep to site **D**? Name any vital structures you know of which would run subcutaneously over this muscle group at **D**. What would be the consequence to a live dog of severance of these structures?

(e) Veterinary surgeons may be seen inserting a hypodermic needle at site **E**. What are they trying to achieve and what precise anatomical structure are they involving in the process?

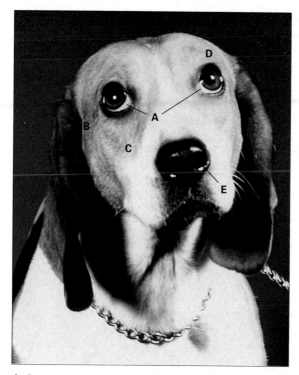

▲ 5.
(a) Identify and name the structures marked **A**. What is their function?
(b) Identify and name the bony area palpable subcutaneously at **B**. What bones of the skull are involved in its anatomical formation?
(c) Identify and name the aperture that might be palpated through the subcutaneous structures found in region **C**. State in which bone of the skull it is situated.
(d) Identify and name the palpable bony protuberance found at **D**. To which bone of the skull does it belong and name any ligamentous structure which might connect it with another bone of the skull? Name that second bone and describe the purpose of the ligament.
(e) Identify and name the aperture indicated by **E**. Name precisely the region of the chamber which lies immediately within this opening.

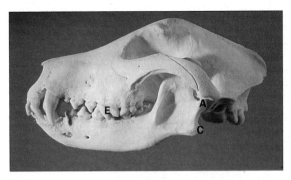

▲ 6.
(a) Name the joint formed at **A** and give its classification.
(b) What structures form the articular surfaces of this joint in life?
(c) Identify prominence **C** and name any muscles which insert onto it.
(d) Give the action of any muscles named in (c) along with their motor nerve supply.
(e) Name tooth **E**, giving the precise name which is associated with its function. To which grouping of teeth does it belong and what characteristics of its root formation conditions the method used for its surgical extraction?

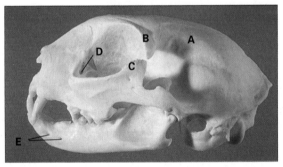

▲ 7.
(a) Name which area of bone bears the marker **A** and state the species to which it belongs. What space does it overlie in life?
(b) Identify and name prominence **B** and state which skull bone it belongs to.
(c) Identify and name prominence **C** and state which skull bone it belongs to. Name any structure which joins **B** and **C** in life.
(d) Name aperture **D** and the skull bone in which it is situated. Is anything found in this space in life? Give details.
(e) Name apertures **E** and the bone in which they are situated. Name anything which passes through them in life.

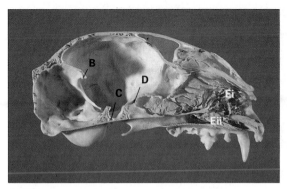

▲ 8.
(a) Identify the species and describe the plane of section which is displayed here.
(b) Identify and name bony structure **B**. State which areas of the brain it separates in life.
(c) Identify and name bony depression **C** and state which neurological structure is located here in the live animal.
(d) Identify the aperture which is marked **D** and state what passes through it in life.
(e) Identify and name the bony areas **Ei** and **Eii** and state which passageways are formed between them in life.

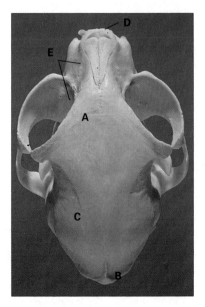

◄9.
(a) Identify and name bone **A**. Which species is this?
(b) Identify and name bone **B**. Of which natural aperture in the skull would this bone form the perimeter?
(c) Identify and name bone **C**. What area of which vital organ would lie deep to this?
(d) Identify and name bone **D**. Which non-bony structures would be found within this bone in life?
(e) Identify and name bone **E**. Is the full extent of this bone displayed here? Give details in your answer.

7

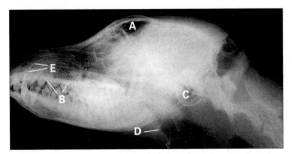

▲ 10.
(a) Identify and name the darkened area at **A** and state which region of the skull it represents. Account for the darkened image produced.
(b) Identify and name the structure imaged at **B**. Which regions of the skull would lie dorsal and ventral to this structure? Give precise names.
(c) Identify the darkened area at **C** and name what particular passageway it represents. Explain why it is imaged as a darkened area.
(d) Identify the fine line imaged at **D** and state what soft tissue structure it is associated with in life.
(e) Identify the structure which is imaged at **E** and state which part of which complete structure it represents. In which bony area of the skull does this structure lie?

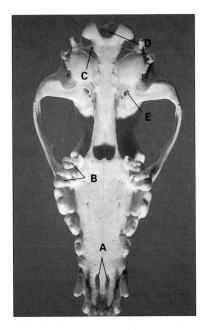

◀ 11.
(a) Identify and name apertures **A** and name the bones of the skull they lie between. Does anything pass through these apertures in life?
(b) Identify and name structures **B**. Classify these structures as they occur within the series of structures lying rostral to them and give an account of their function. In which bone of the skull do they lie and how do they make an attachment within the bone? Give details.
(c) Identify and name aperture **C**. What bone of the skull does it occur in and what passes through it in life?
(d) Identify and name aperture **D**. State what structures might be found passing through it in life.
(e) Identify and name aperture **E**. State what neurological structure might pass through it in life.

12. ▶

(a) Identify and name bone **A**. State the bones of the skull it articulates with (both rostrally and caudally).

(b) Identify and name structures **B**. Which bone of the skull do they belong to?

(c) Identify and name the surfaces marked **C**. Describe anything that makes contact with these surfaces in real life. Which bone of the skull is **C** part of?

(d) Identify and name the portion of bone marked **D** and state to which bone of the skull it belongs.

(e) Identify and name aperture **E** and state in which bone of the skull it is found. What structure is found in this aperture in life? Classify the method of attachment of this structure within the space formed by the aperture.

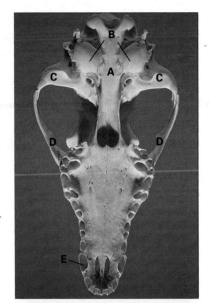

13. ▶

(a) Identify and name bony eminence **A**. Which bone of the skull of what species does it belong to? Which bony structure does it make a close association with in life?

(b) Identify and name bony structure **B**. Name any soft-tissue structures which attach to or run over it in life.

(c) Identify and name aperture **C**. In which bone of the skull does it lie? What neurological structure might be found passing through it in life?

(d) Identify and name structure **D**. State, with reasons, if it falls into the same grouping in the series as the structure lying immediately rostral to it. Does the presence of **D** give any indicator of the age of this cat? Give reasons.

(e) Identify and describe the significance of the coloured line running through the area marked **E**.

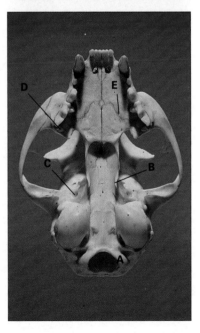

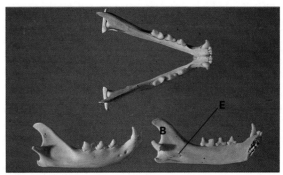

▲ 14.

(a) Identify and name the bones which are present in this photograph.

(b) Name the area of the bone which is marked **B**.

(c) Identify and precisely name the non-bony structures ranged along the dorsal margins of these bones.

(d) In view of your answer to (c), can you identify this species? Give reasons.

(e) Identify and name aperture **E**. Name and describe the origin of any vascular structure which enters at this point.

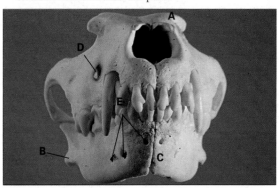

▲ 15.

(a) Identify and name bone **A**. Give the name for the process which can be seen projecting laterally from this bone on either side of the skull.

(b) Identify and name the bone projection **B** and state to which bone it belongs. Name any muscles which attach here in life and give their action and motor nerve supply.

(c) Identify and name region **C**. What type of tissue normally occupies this location in life? Comment on whether this is a feature in all dogs.

(d) Identify and name aperture **D** stating in which bone of the skull it is found. Describe the origins of and name the structures which pass through this aperture in the live dog and indicate which regions they service.

(e) Identify and name apertures **E** stating in which bone they occur. Describe the origins of and name any neurological structures which pass through these apertures in the live dog and indicate which regions they service.

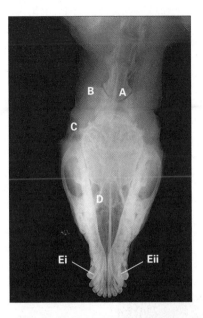

◀ **16.**

(a) Identify and name surface **A** and state to which bone it belongs.

(b) Identify and name area **B** and state to which bone it belongs

(c) Identify and name bony prominence **C** and state to which bone of the skull it belongs.

(d) Identify and name area **D** and state to which bone of the skull it belongs.

(e) Identify and name the type of structures at **Ei** and **Eii**. Distinguish, with reasons, whether **Ei** and **Eii** belong to the upper or lower jaw.

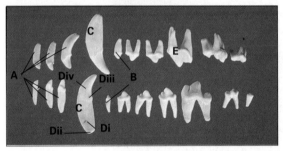

▲ **17.**

(a) Identify and name the type of teeth marked **A**. Describe where they are located in the skull in life.

(b) Identify and name the teeth marked **B**. Do these teeth belong to the temporary or permanent dentition?

(c) Identify and name the teeth marked **C**. What is their function? In life, which of these teeth lies most rostrally when the mouth is closed, the upper or the lower?

(d) Give the correct regional names for the areas of the tooth marked **Di**, **Dii**, **Diii** and **Div** and describe the tissue types either covering or associated with these surfaces.

(e) Describe the function of tooth **E** giving its specialised name and its correct placement in the serial row of upper teeth. With which surface does it make contact with in the lower row of teeth? If there was abcessation of the roots of this tooth where would you expect the swelling caused to manifest itself in the live dog?

11

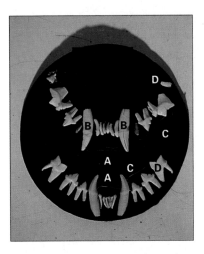

◀ **18.**
(a) Identify and name the group of teeth marked **A**.
(b) Identify and name the group of teeth marked **B**.
(c) Identify and name the group of teeth marked **C**.
(d) Identify and name the group of teeth marked **D**.
(e) From the information given in (a) to (d) identify the species and age group involved here, giving reasons for your selection.

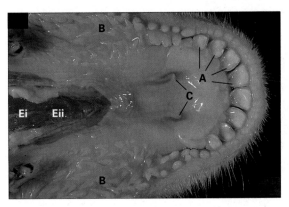

▲ **19.**
(a) Identify and name the structures which are marked **A** and comment if they can all be classified as belonging to the same type.
(b) Identify and name the regions which are marked **B** and classify the structures which are seen lying on their surfaces.
(c) Identify and name the structures which are marked **C** and state what openings may be found upon them.
(d) Using the criteria seen in the previous answers, identify the type of species shown giving reasons for your answer.
(e) A radical resection of an organ has been made at **Ei**. Name the resected organ and identify the muscle which has been cut through at **Eii** to perform the removal.

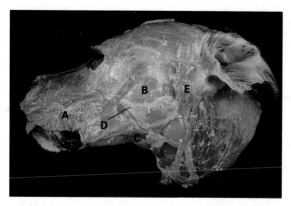

▲ 20.
(a) Identify and name the area of muscle **A** and give an indication of its function.
(b) Identify and name muscle **B** and give its origins and insertions.
(c) Identify and name muscle **C** and give its origins and insertions.
(d) Identify and name nerve trunk **D**. Give the parent trunk of this nerve. If this parent trunk were to be completely severed, would it affect all or some of muscles **A**, **B** and **C**? Give details to accompany your answer.
(e) Identify and name the structure marked **E**. What is its collective function and describe in detail any connections it makes with more rostrally placed head regions.

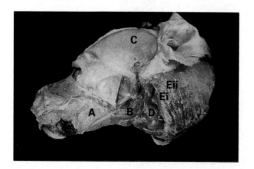

▲ 21.
(a) Identify and name muscle **A**. State what its function is when it contracts and give its motor nerve supply.
(b) Identify and name muscle **B**. State its action and give its motor nerve supply.
(c) Identify and name muscle **C**. State the action of this muscle and give its motor nerve supply.
(d) Identify the group of muscles to which **D** belongs and, if possible, name muscle **D**. State its function and give the motor nerve supply.
(e) **Ei** and **Eii** mark the heads of origin of which collective muscle? State the points of attachment of this muscle and describe its action, giving the motor nerve supply.

13

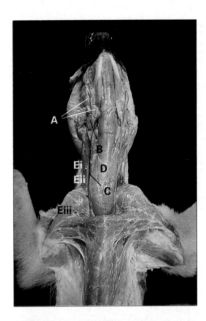

◀ **22.**
(a) Identify and name the structures marked **A** giving topographical reasons for your choice of answer.
(b) Identify and name structure **B** giving topographical reasons for your choice of answer.
(c) Identify and name vessel **C**. Describe and name the vessels forming it rostrally and indicate how it terminates caudally.
(d) Identify and name muscle **D** giving its origin and insertion. What is the function of the muscle?
(e) Identify muscles **Ei**, **Eii** and **Eiii** and describe how they are interrelated. What is their collective function and motor nerve supply?

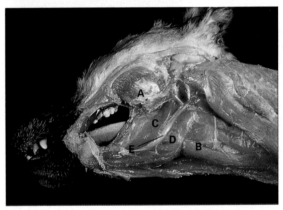

▲ **23.**
(a) Identify and name the muscle which has been cut at **A** to allow removal of the mandible.
(b) Identify and name muscle **B** and state its action.
(c) Identify and name muscle **C** and state its action.
(d) Identify and name muscle **D** and state its action.
(e) Identify and name structure **E**. If structure **E** was totally sectioned which of the previous structures **A** to **D** would be affected? Give reasons for your answer.

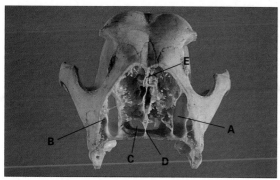

▲ 24.

(a) Identify and name space **A**.

(b) Identify and name space **B** and state what structures might be found occupying it in life.

(c) Identify and name space **C** and state which bone of the skull forms its ventral margin. What further space does **C** communicate with caudally?

(d) Identify and name bone **D** and state which collective structure it belongs to.

(e) Identify and name skull bone **E**. Name two further regions of this bone which can also be seen on this section.

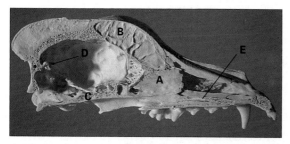

▲ 25.

(a) Identify and name area **A** and state which bone of the skull it belongs to. This structure appears incomplete rostrally; is this the case in real life or can you describe, giving details, a rostral continuation that might be present normally?

(b) Identify and name area **B** and state which bone it belongs to. Does the presence of this area tell you anything about the plane of section? Give reasons for your answer.

(c) Identify and name area **C** and state which bone it belongs to. Name the bony area immediately dorsal to the marker and state what soft tissue structure would lie in close association with this area in life.

(d) Identify and name the area of bone marked **D** and state which bone it belongs to. This bony area can be seen to project rostrally. Can you name, precisely, any soft tissue structures that it comes into apposition with in life as it projects rostrally?

(e) Identify bone **E** and state with which other bones of the skull it joins in the adult dog.

15

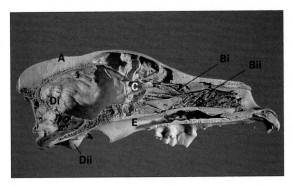

▲ 26.
(a) Identify and name bone **A**. How would you classify this type of bone and what region of which vital soft tissue structure does it overlie in life?

(b) Identify and name structures **Bi** and **Bii**. State what space lies between them in life.

(c) Identify and name region **C**. State which bone it belongs to. Indicate which region of which soft tissue structure is associated with the caudal face of region **C**.

(d) Name the areas of bone marked **Di** and **Dii**. Are these two areas part of the same bone or are they derived from different sources? Give names with your answer.

(e) Identify and name the passageway indicated by **E**. What soft tissue structure would control flow through this passageway in life and where would it lie relative to **E**?

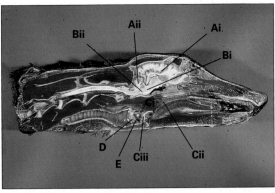

▲ 27.
(a) Identify and name regions **Ai** and **Aii**.

(b) Identify and name regions **Bi** and **Bii**.

(c) Name region **Ci** and identify structures **Cii** and **Ciii** which appear to form the floor of the region.

(d) Identify and name the fold of tissue marked **D** and state the structures or regions it attaches to both dorsally and ventrally.

(e) Identify opening **E** and name what it leads into in this region.

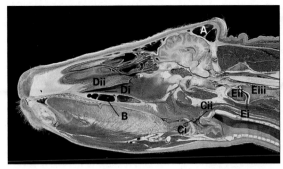

▲ 28.
(a) Identify and name the space which marker **A** is indicating. In which bone of the skull is it situated?
(b) Identify and name the space which marker **B** is indicating. In which bone of the skull is it situated?
(c) Identify and name the space which lies between the markers **Ci** and **Cii**. Which structures demarcate its boundaries?
(d) Identify and name the space to which the marker **Di** is pointing. Which structure is lying dorsal to it at **Dii**?
(e) Identify and name the space marked **Ei**. What lies immediately cranial and caudal to it, marked **Eii** and **Eiii**?

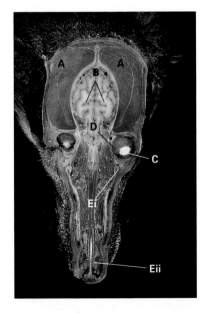

◀ 29.
(a) Identify and name the muscle group marked **A** which has been sectioned. State its function and give the motor nerve supply.
(b) Identify and name the region of the structure marked **B**. Explain the variation of colour in the cut surface.
(c) Identify and name structure **C**. Describe how it is maintained in this position in real life.
(d) Identify and name region **D** and describe what occupies this location in life.
(e) There are openings of a duct system indicated by **Ei** and **Eii**. State what this duct system represents and describe its function.

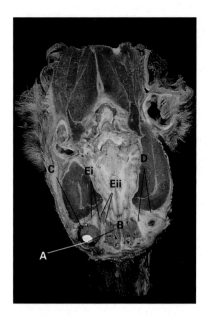

◀ 30.

(a) Identify and name the portion of the eyeball marked **A** and state what tissue layer covers its most rostral surface in life, giving a precise name for this layer.

(b) Name the space indicated by marker **B** and describe what fills this space in life.

(c) Identify and name the outer layer of the eyeball marked **C**. Give a name for the region of the junction of **C** with **A**.

(d) Identify and name the structure forming the surfaces marked **D**. Of what type of tissue is **D** formed and which cavity of the skull does it line?

(e) Name the muscular structures marked **Ei** and **Eii** and in general terms describe what actions they bring about when they contract. Do **Ei** and **Eii** have the same motor nerve supply? Explain your answer.

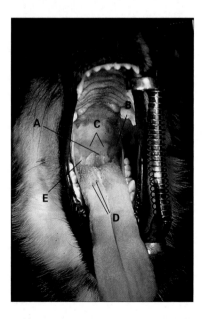

◀ 31.

(a) Identify and name structure **A**. Describe the nature of the tissue which forms **A** and state which larger structure it forms a part of.

(b) Identify and name structure **B** and describe its general function and composition.

(c) Identify and name structure **C** and describe the passageways that it is related to caudally.

(d) Name the organ and its surface as indicated by **D**. The leader lines are indicating specific rounded structures on this surface. Name and attribute them with a function.

(e) Identify and name the fold of tissue running dorsoventrally, indicated by **E**. There are small pointed elevated structures present on the surface at the ventral end of this fold. Name them and state their function.

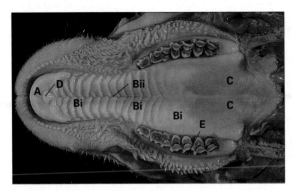

▲ 32.

(a) Identify and name region **A**. Give your reasons for allocating a species type to this specimen.

(b) Identify and name region **Bi** and state which bones of the skull lie deep to it. What is the term for the line marked **Bii**?

(c) Identify and name region **C** and state what structure the caudal edge of this region is closely related to in the live animal.

(d) Identify and name structure **D** and state what opens onto it in life.

(e) Identify and name space **E**. State what structures mark its medial and lateral boundaries and suggest the names of any glandular structures which might open into it in the live animal.

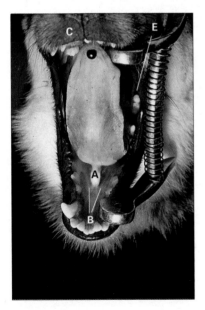

◄ 33.

(a) Identify and name tissue fold **A**. Name the topographical areas and organs it connects.

(b) Identify and name the elevated structure found at **B**. Name any apertures which can be found on **B** indicating what may travel via these apertures in life.

(c) How would you name the region indicated by **C**? What muscle groups would form its deeper layers?

(d) What would be the motor nerve supply to the muscle layer named in (c)? Would the superficial covering and the mucosal lining of that area have sensory innervation via the same nerve trunk? Explain your answer giving specific names of nerves involved.

(e) Identify and name the tooth which lies adjacent to **E**. What name would be given to the area lying lateral to this tooth and what would be the muscle layer forming its lateral boundary?

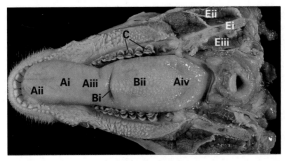

▲ 34.

(a) Identify and name organ **Ai** and the regions of that organ which are marked **Aii**, **Aiii** and **Aiv**.

(b) Identify and name folded area **Bi**. Immediately caudal to this are elevations of the surface covering marked **Bii**. What are they termed?

(c) Identify and name the type of structures which are indicated by **C**. Comment on the surface colouration of these structures giving reasons for their appearance.

(d) Using the criteria seen in the previous answers, state your reasons for identifying this species.

(e) Identify and name the bony structure which has been sawn through at **Ei**. Which muscles have also been cut at the level of **Eii** and **Eiii**?

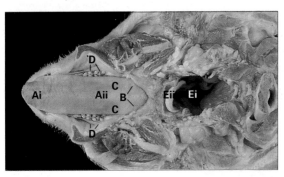

▲ 35.

(a) Identify and name the organ and the regions of that organ marked **Ai** and **Aii**.

(b) The markers **B** are pointing to specific structures which can be seen on the organ surface. What are these structures called?

(c) The markers **C** are pointing to specific regions on the organ surface which have an irregular furrowed appearance. What are the structures called which lie in these regions?

(d) Identify and name the structures marked **D**. Give their classification and type. Using the criteria seen in this and the previous answers, state your reasons for identifying the species.

(e) Identify and name opening **Ei** and state what structure lies at its ventral edge marked **Eii**.

20

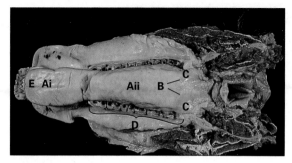

▲ 36.
(a) Identify and name the organ and the region of that organ which are marked **Ai** and **Aii**, respectively.
(b) The markers **B** are pointing at specific structures which are present on the surface of the organ. Name them.
(c) The markers **C** are pointing to specific areas which have a furrowed appearance. State which structures give this appearance. Using the criteria seen in this and previous answers, state your reasons for identifying the species.
(d) Name and classify the structures marked **D**.
(e) Name and classify the structures marked **E**. Comment on the appearance of their visible surfaces. Using the criteria seen in answers (d) and (e) give an approximate age to this animal, giving your reasons.

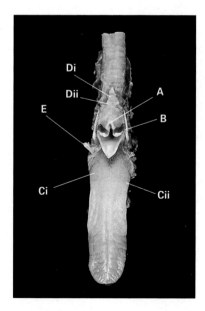

◀ 37.
(a) Identify prominence **A** and state which structure it belongs to.
(b) Identify structure **B**. Name any articulations that it makes with other structures in the region.
(c) The markers **Ci** and **Cii** indicate structures on the tongue's surface. Can you name them and detail their appearance as they are seen in the live dog? State their relative functions.
(d) The tissue remnant **Di** represents a portion of an organ which lay in this dorsal position in life. Name it and state what the organ entrance would be called as it lies in position **Dii**.
(e) This severed structure **E** is composed of bone. What bone complex did it belong to and what region of the skull would this complex be associated with in the live dog?

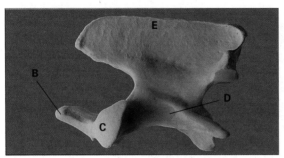

▲ 38.

(a) Identify this bone and name it precisely giving the species. State which group of bones it belongs to and indicate at which position in this group it is normally found.

(b) Identify and name promontory **B**. Indicate which topographical position it occupies in life. What soft tissue structure helps to maintain this promontory in its correct anatomical position in life? If there was excessive movement of structure **B** what soft tissue structures might it come into contact with and what may possibly result?

(c) Identify surface **C** and indicate which area of which bone it approximates to in life. What movements may occur between these surfaces. How would they be classified?

(d) Identify and name aperture **D**. Indicate the name of anything that passes through it in life.

(e) Identify and name promontory **E** and name any ligamentous structure which is closely related to it in life. What is the predominant tissue characteristic of this structure? Indicate where you would search to palpate **E** in a live animal.

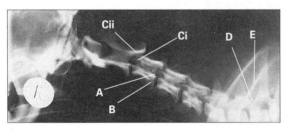

▲ 39.

(a) Identify and name the darkened area **A**. What soft tissue structure would be found at this area in life? Be precise in your description.

(b) Identify the darkened area **B** stating what soft tissue structure would be found at this area in life.

(c) Identify the darkened line between markers **Ci** and **Cii** and state what this represents in life.

(d) Identify and name bone **D**. Give its precise location and number in the sequence of bones to which it belongs. Give two bony features that would verify your choice of answer.

(e) Identify and name structure **E**. Explain why it is imaged as such a densely white structure compared with the other bony projection it crosses over.

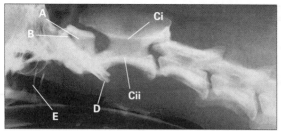

▲ 40.

(a) Identify and name the region seen in this radiograph indicating the angle of projection. Is the left edge of the plate cranial or caudal? Name bone **A**.

(b) Identify and name the darkened area **B** and name what this image represents in life. Name anything which passes through area **B** in life.

(c) Identify and name the area between **Ci** and **Cii**. Name what this image represents in life. What soft tissue structures are found running through this area in life?

(d) Identify structure **D** and indicate where this may be found on palpation in life.

(e) Identify structure **E** and name what this image represents in real life. Name any muscle which might connect **E** with a major mobile organ of the head region. State what action this muscle might have.

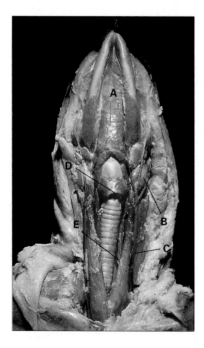

◀ 41.

(a) Identify and name muscle **A**. Give the name which is applied to the way in which the muscles of **A** meet in the midline. What is the muscle action during contraction and what is the underlying motor nerve supply?

(b) Identify and name **B**. Name the vessels which can be seen lying both lateral and medial to it.

(c) Name **C**. Identify the muscular bands which can be seen lying on either side.

(d) Identify and name **D** describing which portion is visible. Name the muscle bundles which attach to **D** immediate to each side of the midline. What is the nerve supply and where does this nerve trunk derive from? Is this nerve origin typical of other muscles in the immediate region? Discuss your answer giving names.

(e) The marker **E** indicates a band-like collection of structures running the length of the cervical region. Name it and its component parts, indicating their direction of travel.

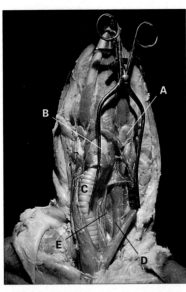

(a) Identify and name structure **A**. indicating its function and regional significance.

(b) Identify prominence **B** and the structure which it belongs to. Explain how this elevation is formed.

(c) Identify structure **C** and describe the configuration of the various types of tissues which constitute this collective structure.

(d) Identify and name structure **D** and indicate the topographical position of its origin and termination. What type of tissue forms the major component of its wall?

(e) Identify and name muscle **E**. If this muscle was loosened from its bony attachments and elevated laterally at this position what structures might be revealed deep to it?

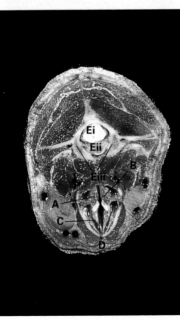

◀ 43.

(a) Identify and name cartilaginous structures **A** and state which collective structure they belong to.

(b) Identify and name muscular body **B** and state its action on contraction indicating the motor nerve supply involved. What is the source of this nerve trunk?

(c) Identify and name the band-like strip of tissue **C**. State what it attaches to both dorsally and ventrally. What are its component structures?

(d) The structures **C** lie to either side of the midline. What name is given to the space created between them at **D**? Would this space be of constant width in the live dog or would there be variations? Explain your answer giving the functional anatomy of that region.

(e) Remembering the level of this section, identify and name structures **Ei**, **Eii** and **Eiii**. Elaborate on the potential problems of their close proximity and state what anatomical structures assist in controlling this situation.

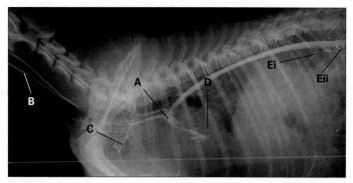

▲ 44.
(a) Identify and name the vessel imaged at **A** and state its point of origin.
(b) Identify and name the vessel imaged at **B**. Describe the areas this vessel supplies and verify, giving names and position on this radiograph, if there is any alternative supply to the areas you have described.
(c) Identify and name the vessel imaged at **C** and state what major region this vessel supplies and describe the course it takes to achieve this supply.
(d) Identify and name the fine vessel imaged at **D** and indicate the organ it supplies. Describe the point of origin of this vessel giving topographical detail.
(e) Identify and name the vessels marked **Ei** and **Eii** and detail which organs each vessel supplies.

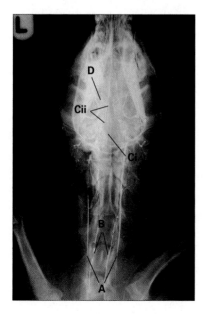

◀ 45.
(a) Identify and name the vessels marked **A** and state their origin.
(b) Identify and name the vessels marked **B** and state their origin.
(c) Identify and name vessel **Ci** and indicate the name of the composite vascular structure **Cii** it is flowing towards and to which it contributes.
(d) Name vessel **D** which is flowing from **Cii**.
(e) Relate the location of structure **Cii** to recognisable landmarks of the brain, giving their names.

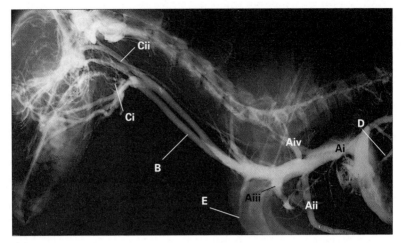

▲ 46.

(a) Identify the vessel marked **Ai** and name its major contributories marked **Aii**, **Aiii** and **Aiv**.

(b) Identify vessel **B** and state which major area it drains.

(c) Identify and name the vessels marked **Ci** and **Cii** and describe any glandular structures which can be found at their site of confluence in life.

(d) Identify and name vessel **D** and state which location it normally drains into.

(e) Identify and name vessel **E** and describe its region of drainage.

Thoracic Limb

47. ▶

(a) Identify and give the anatomical term to describe region **A**. Which is the major bone of this region?

(b) Identify and give the anatomical term to describe region **B**. What are the major bones of this region? How would you describe this aspect of the limb and what would be the term used to describe the opposite surface.

(c) Identify and give the anatomical term to describe region **C**. What are the major bones of this region? How would you describe this aspect of the limb and what would be the term used to describe the opposite surface?

(d) Identify and name structure **D** and state the bone which it is most closely related to.

(e) Identify and name region **E** and state which part of which bone it is most closely related to.

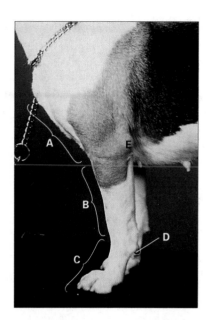

48. ▶

(a) Identify and name the joint which lies at region **A** and state the articular surfaces involved.

(b) Identify and name the muscle which can be seen running beneath the skin surface at **B**. What is the action of the muscle on **A** and where is it inserting relative to **A**?

(c) Identify and name the joint which lies at region **C** and state the articular surfaces involved. List the range of movements normally experienced at this joint in the live animal.

(d) Identify and name structures **Di** and **Dii**. Do both of these structures contain exactly the same bony elements? Explain your answer giving names

(e) A major vessel lies subcutaneously at **E**. Name it and state its clinical significance. Are there any neurological structures also related to **E** which the clinician should be aware of? Give names with your answer.

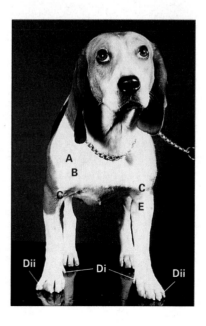

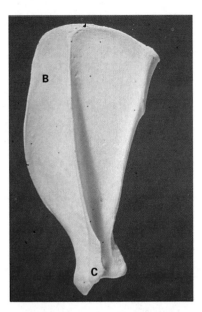

◀ 49.
(a) Identify this bone and state which limb it originates from. Name the species and level of maturity of this animal giving suitable reasons for your choice.
(b) Name the area marked **B** and indicate what structure would be adherent to it in life.
(c) Identify the structure marked **C** and name any muscle which attaches here.
(d) Name any other attachments of this muscle and describe its action stating which joint it affects.
(e) What would be the motor nerve supply to the muscle in (d)? If this major trunk were damaged could you describe any areas of concurrent loss of sensation that might be detected?

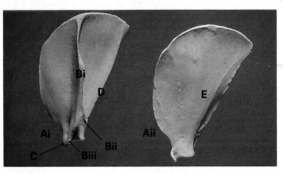

▲ 50.
(a) Identify and name this bone. Indicate which aspect of the bone is represented in **Ai** and **Aii**.
(b) Identify the structures marked **Bi**, **Bii** and **Biii**. Do any of these structures help you to identify the species. Give reasons for your selection.
(c) Identify the region of the bone marked **C** and state which muscle would attach here in life. Where would its other attachment lie?
(d) Identify the region of the bone marked **D** and state which muscle would attach here in life. Where would its other attachment lie?
(e) Identify and name the region marked **E** and state which muscle would attach here in life. Where would its other attachments lie?

51. ▶

(a) Identify and name the type of bone displayed and state which aspect of it is shown at **A**.

(b) Orientate this bone by naming the borders and angles which are marked **Bi**, **Bii**, **Biii** and **Biv**.

(c) Identify and name structure **Ci** and give the term for the prominent part of it marked **Cii**.

(d) Identify and name prominence **D** and state the name of a structure which attaches here in the live animal.

(e) Using the criteria seen in the previous answers, identify this species giving reasons for your choice.

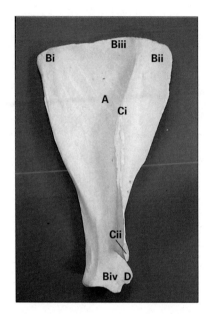

52. ▶

(a) Identify and name the type of bone displayed and, with reasons, whether it is from a left or right limb.

(b) Identify and name border **B** and comment on the irregular appearance of the edge.

(c) Identify and name structure **C**.

(d) Identify and name the region of the bone, the periphery of which is marked **D**.

(e) Using the criteria seen in the previous answers, identify the species giving reasons.

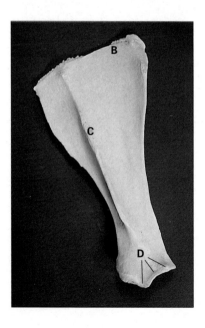

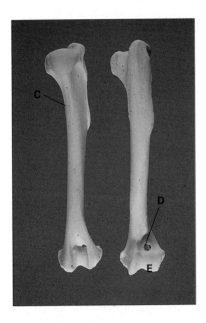

◀ **53.**
(a) Identify this bone and name the species, giving three major reasons for your choice of species.
(b) Which aspect is seen of the bone on the left, and which limb does the bone belong to?
(c) Name structure **C** and state what attaches here in real life.
(d) Name aperture **D** and indicate any structures you know which pass through this space in life.
(e) Name precisely the area marked **E** and indicate which area of which bone this articulates with in life.

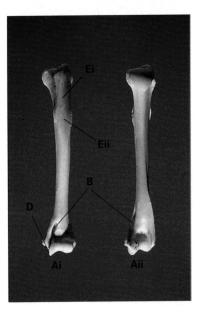

◀ **54.**
(a) Identify these bones and state whether the bones **Ai** and **Aii** are from the right or left leg of the animal.
(b) Identify and name the apertures marked **B** and describe how their presence might assist in identifying the species.
(c) Relate any structures that you know of which pass through the apertures marked **B**.
(d) Identify and name the region of bone marked **D** and state which part of which bone it is related to in the live animal.
(e) Identify and name the regions of bone marked **Ei** and **Eii** and state which muscles insert onto or originate from these regions.

55. ▶
(a) Identify and name the type of bone displayed here.
(b) Identify and name the region of the bone which is marked **B**.
(c) Identify and name the region of the bone which is marked **C**.
(d) Identify and name the region of the bone which is marked **D**.
(e) Using the criteria seen in the previous answers, state your reasons for identifying the species and whether this bone is from a left or right limb.

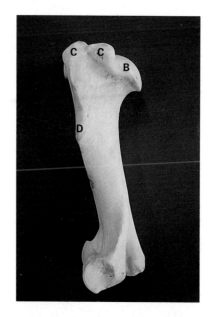

56. ▶
(a) Identify and name the type of bone displayed here.
(b) Identify and name the region of the bone marked **B**.
(c) Identify and name the region of the bone marked **C**.
(d) Identify and name the regions of the bone marked **Di** and **Dii**.
(e) Using the criteria seen in the previous answers, name, giving reasons, the species and whether this bone is from the left or right limb.

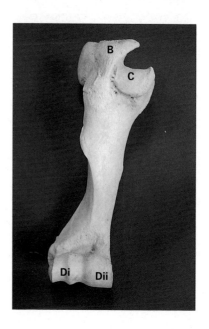

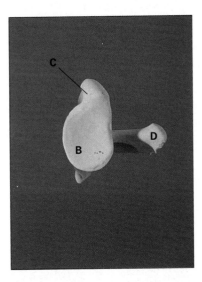

◄57.
(a) Name the bone and identify the aspect under view in this photograph.
(b) Name area **B** and state what type of tissue covers and surrounds this surface in life.
(c) Identify and name bone projection **C**. In which direction does this project in the live animal?
(d) Identify and name projection **D**. In which direction does this project in the live animal?
(e) Name any muscle tendons of the region that run in the area between **B** and **D**.

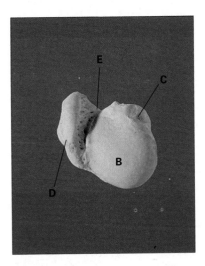

◄58.
(a) Name the bone and the aspect of the bone which is viewed in this photograph.
(b) Identify and name region **B** and state to which part of which bone it is closely related to in life.
(c) Identify and name bony projection **C** and state on which side of the bone it is found in life.
(d) Identify and name bony projection **D** and name the muscles which attach here.
(e) Identify and name the depression on the bone surface marked **E** and describe any structures which are found running in this area in life.

59. ▶
(a) Name the bone and the aspect of the bone which is being viewed in this photograph.
(b) Identify and name the area of bone marked **B** and state which area of which bone it is closely associated with in the live animal.
(c) Identify and name the area of bone marked **C** and state which area of which bone it is closely associated with in life.
(d) Identify and name the bony recess marked **D** and state on which aspect of the bone it is found in the live animal.
(e) What bony structure is found in close proximity to area **D** in the live animal?

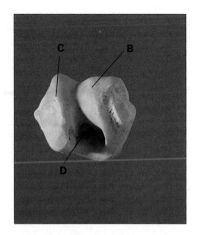

60. ▶
(a) The markers **Ai** and **Aii** have a black line running in the area between them and there is also a black line running in the area immediately distal and cranial to the marker **Aii**. What is the significance of these lines and do they represent the same structures?
(b) Identify and name promontory **B** and indicate the significance of the black line running cranial to it. Do you think this might be a fracture?
(c) Identify and name the bones marked **Ci** and **Cii** and state how they are held in position relative to each other.
(d) Identify and name the region of the bone marked **D** and state whether this area has a similar appearance at all stages in the life of the animal.
(e) In the area marked **E** the images are of different shades of near white, grey and near black. Can you explain this variation in image colour in the immediate area of the marker, both distal and cranial to it?

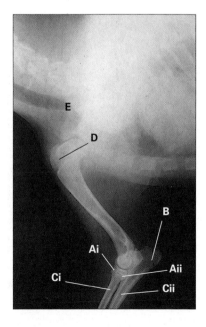

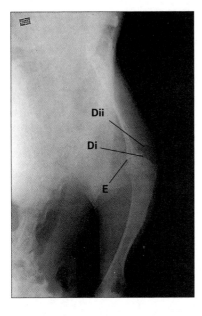

◀ 61.

(a) Identify and name the joint imaged in the centre of the field. Classify and describe the normal movements.

(b) Describe the angle of projection and indicate the orientation of the limb by stating which side of the plate represents the most lateral structures. Give three prominent bony features of the limb to substantiate your answer.

(c) Name both lateral and medially placed soft tissue structures which are responsible for limiting this joint to its normal range of movement.

(d) Name the major nerve trunk that travels in the space between **Di** and **Dii**. Does this trunk travel cranially or caudally to the joint when passing from medial to lateral? Explain how damage to the trunk might interfere with joint stability.

(e) Identify surface **E**. What nature of tissue covers this surface? Is this radiographic image a true representation of the complete extent of this surface in the live animal? Explain.

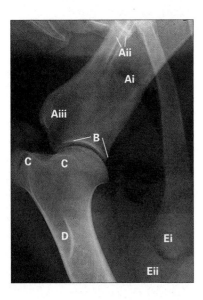

◀ 62.

(a) Identify and name the bone and the regions of that bone which are marked **Ai**, **Aii** and **Aiii**.

(b) Identify and name the area which is defined by markers **B**. Of which structure does it form a part?

(c) Identify and name the bone and the regions of that bone marked **C**. Using the criteria seen in this and previous answers, state your reasons for identifying the species.

(d) Identify and name the structure which is creating the image marked **D**.

(e) Identify and name the bones which are marked **Ei** and **Eii**.

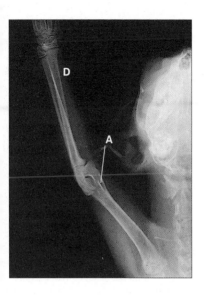

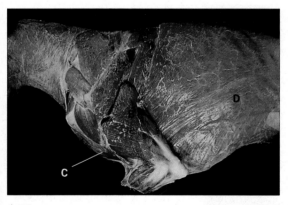

◀ 63.
(a) Name aperture **A** and identify which bone it lies in.
(b) Does the presence of this aperture help identify the species? If so, which species is it? Are there any other bony features associated with this limb which would support your choice?
(c) Name any structures which pass through aperture **A** in life.
(d) There are two bony shafts present at level **D** in the limb. Name them and indicate which of them lies in the more lateral position.
(e) At the distal end of the lateral bone there appears to be a separate bony element. Is this a normal feature in this species and, if so, what is this structure termed?

▲ 64.
(a) Name muscle **A**. What is its function and its motor nerve supply?
(b) Name muscle **B**. What is its function and its motor nerve supply?
(c) Name muscle **C**. What is its function and its motor nerve supply?
(d) Name muscle **D**. What is its function and its motor nerve supply?
(e) If there was a complete tear of the brachial plexus which of these muscles would lose its motor nerve supply? Give reasons for each muscle in your reply.

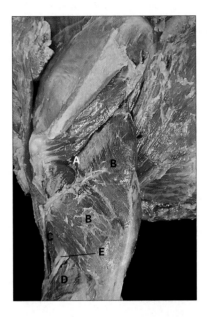

◀ 65.

(a) Identify and name muscle **A**. What is the action of this muscle when it contracts? Which aspect of which joint space does it overlie?

(b) Identify and name muscle **B**. What is the action of this muscle when it contracts?

(c) Identify and name muscle **C**. What is the action of this muscle when it contracts?

(d) Identify and name muscle **D**. What is the action of this muscle when it contracts?

(e) Identify nerve trunk **E**. If this trunk were to be accidently severed at this point in a live dog, which of the muscles **A** to **D** would remain functional and which would cease to contract voluntarily?

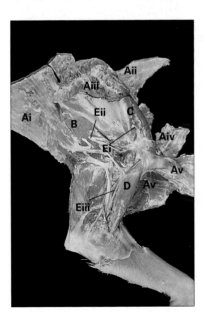

◀ 66.

(a) The limb has been resected from the trunk by section of a series of muscles. State which aspect of the limb is being viewed here and identify the resected muscles marked **Ai, Aii, Aiii, Aiv** and **Av**.

(b) Identify and name muscle **B** and state its origin, insertion and action.

(c) Identify and name muscle **C** and state its origin, insertion and action.

(d) Identify and name muscle **D** and state its origin, insertion and action.

(e) The markers **Ei, Eii** and **Eiii** are indicating nerve trunks running in the limb. Identify and name these trunks and match each of them in terms of motor supply with one of the muscles marked **B, C** and **D**.

67. ▶
(a) Identify and name these bones.
Indicate which aspects are being
viewed in **Ai** and **Aii**.
(b) Identify and name the surface areas of
bone marked **Bi** and **Bii** and state
which parts of which other bones are
closely associated with them in the live
animal.
(c) Identify and name promontory **C** and
indicate the structures which attach to
the bone in this position.
(d) Identify and name bony projection **D**
and state which side of the bone this is
found on in the live animal.
(e) There is a small perforation in the
bone at **E**. Can you name what it
represents and indicate what type of
structures would be passing through it
in life?

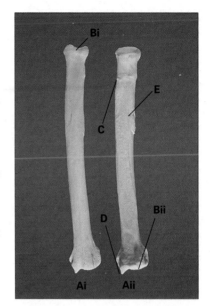

68. ▶
(a) Identify the bone with species, giving
reasons for your choice. Name
structure **A**. Which area or space is
this structure related to in the normal
standing animal?
(b) Identify and name structure **B**. Which
area, of which structure, is **B** closely
related to in the normal standing
animal?
(c) Identify and name structure **C**. Name
the attachments made to this structure
in life.
(d) Identify and name structure **D**. In life
does this structure articulate with any
other surfaces? If so, name them.
(e) In a live animal in the normal standing
position, which of the structures **A** to
D can be readily palpated subcutaneously? Which are non-palpable?

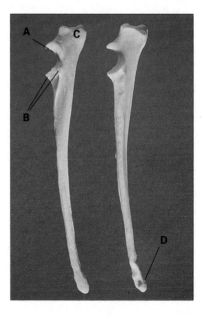

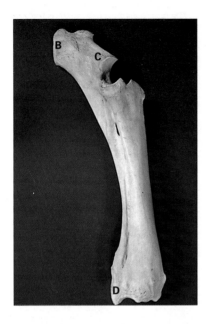

(a) Identify and name the types of bones displayed here.
(b) Identify and name the region of bone marked **B**. Of which bone is it a part?
(c) Identify and name the region of bone marked **C** and state with which area of which bone it is closely related in the live animal.
(d) Identify and name the region of bone marked **D**.
(e) Using the criteria seen in the previous answers, name, giving reasons, the species and which aspect of the bones are shown.

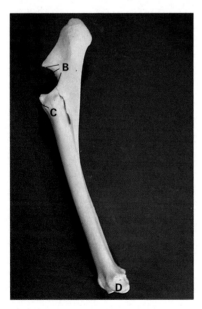

◀ 70.
(a) Identify and name the types of bones displayed here.
(b) State the term used to describe the region, the outline of which is indicated by the markers **B**. Of which bone does it form a part?
(c) Identify and name the raised portion of bone marked **C** and state what attaches here in the live animal.
(d) Identify and name the region of bone marked **D** and state which bone it is a part of.
(e) Using the criteria seen in the previous answers, name, giving reasons, the species and whether these bones come from a right or left limb. Does the knowledge of species affect your answers to the latter part of question (d)? Explain your answers.

71. ▶

(a) Identify the region and the species being imaged and describe the projection of the radiograph.

(b) Identify and explain the significance of the dark line which is marked **B**.

(c) Identify and explain the significance of the dark line marked **C**. The activity of which structures might alter the shape and position of the image marked at **C**?

(d) Identify and name the white densely imaging structure seen at **D**.

(e) Identify and name the promontories marked **Ei** and **Eii**. In the live animal on which aspect of the bone does each of them lie? Give reasons for your answer.

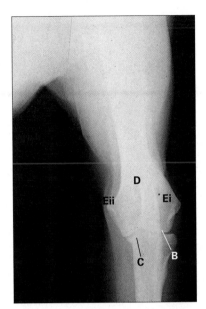

72. ▶

(a) Identify the region and species shown. Which aspect is shown? Is this from the left or right side of the animal?

(b) Using the number of specific bones present, how would you classify this species as to its mode of stance and weight bearing?

(c) Identify and name bone **Ci** and give the term for the ridge marked **Cii**, stating what type of tissue or structure is associated with it in the live animal.

(d) In life, region **Di** is converted into a canal-like structure by a layer of tissue extending from **Dii** to **Diii**. What is this layer termed? Which tendinous structures will pass through this canal?

(e) In life areas **Ei**, **Eii** and **Eiii** are converted into smooth passageways to allow tendinous structures to pass over them. What terms are given to these areas and which tendons run past each of them? What holds these tendons in place?

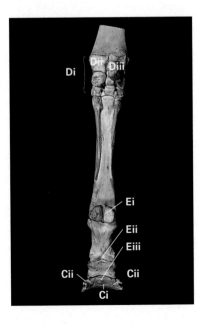

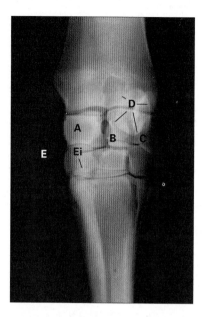

◀73.

(a) State which region is under study and which species it belongs to. Identify and name the bone over which marker **A** lies.

(b) Identify and name the bone over which marker **B** lies.

(c) Identify and name the bone over which marker **C** lies.

(d) Identify and name the bone which is outlined by the markers **D**.

(e) The marker **Ei** is indicating a small radiodense area overlying a larger area. Explain and name what is being imaged here. Does marker **E** lie to the medial or lateral side of this region? Give reasons for your answer.

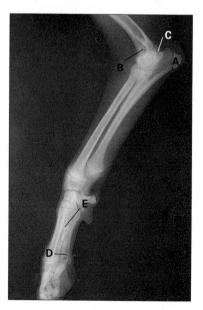

◀74.

(a) Identify and name prominence **A** which appears to be a piece of bone separated from the adjacent main bony body. Is this a true statement of the condition in life? Please comment.

(b) Identify the darker area of reduced radio-opacity **B** and give a name to this area. Is this a constant feature of a normal dog limb?

(c) Identify the region of reduced radio-opacity **C** and name what region it represents in real life. Is this a constant feature of a normal dog limb?

(d) Identify area **D** and state whether it belongs to the bony body, or lies proximal or distal to it. Give reasons for your choice. Is the appearance of **D** a constant feature of a normal dog limb?

(e) Identify the area of reduced radio-opacity **E**. Name the structure it represents in life. Is this area a constant feature of a normal dog limb?

75. ▶
(a) Identify and name what is represented by the dark line marked **A**.
(b) Identify and name what is represented by the dark line marked **B**.
(c) Identify and name what is represented by the dark line marked **C**.
(d) Identify and name what is represented by the dark line marked **D**.
(e) Identify and name what is represented by the dark line marked **E**. Compare and contrast the types of tissues which are involved at **A** to **E**.

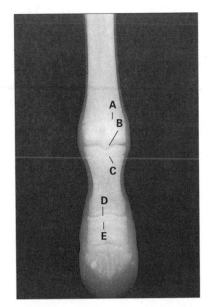

76. ▶
(a) Identify and name promontory **A**. Which bone is it part of and which ligament of which joint attaches here?
(b) Identify and name muscle **B**. What is the action of this muscle? State its motor nerve supply.
(c) Identify and name muscle **C**. What is the action of this muscle? State its motor nerve supply.
(d) If the major nerve trunks to muscles **B** and **C** were severed would there be concurrent loss of cutaneous sensation in the distal limb? If so, describe the areas affected for each nerve trunk under separate headings for **B** and **C**.
(e) Identify and name vessel **E**. In which direction is the blood travelling through this vessel and where are its connections with the major blood vessels of the neck and trunk?

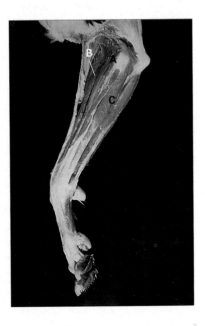

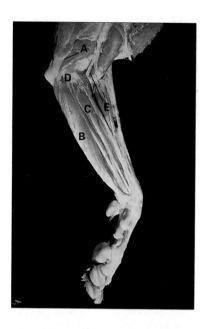

◀77.
(a) Identify the region of the specimen which occupies the centre of this photograph and lies distal to **A**. Indicate which aspect of the specimen is being viewed. Give the name of muscle **A**.
(b) Identify and name muscle **B**.
(c) Identify and name muscle **C**.
(d) Identify and name the prominent feature marked **D** and state if it would be palpable in the live animal. It is noticeable that the muscles **B** and **C** originate from **D**. Does this assist in confirming their actions? Explain your answer and give the appropriate actions for each muscle.
(e) A nerve trunk is marked at **E**. Identify and name it. Comment on whether it would be responsible for innervating any of the muscles named above.

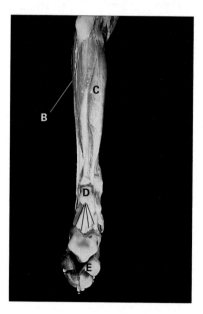

◀78.
(a) Given that this is the caudal aspect, is this a left or right limb? Give reasons using two bony landmarks.
(b) Identify and name muscle **B**. What is the action of this muscle? State its motor nerve supply.
(c) Identify and name muscle **C**. What is the action of this muscle? State its motor nerve supply.
(d) Identify and name the structures marked **D**. On which bone and at what precise level do these structures terminate?
(e) Name structure **E**. What is its function and how does its composition assist it to act as such? If the dog were to sustain a severe penetrating laceration of this structure, what essential structures might also be affected and what would be the result on the overall action of the toe?

79. ▶

(a) Identify and name the region which is displayed in the centre of this photograph and state which aspect of the region is being viewed in **Ai** and **Aii**.

(b) Identify and name each of the following bones: **Bi**, **Bii** and **Biii**. How do these bones develop in the young animal?

(c) Identify and name the bones marked **Ci**, **Cii**, **Ciii** and **Civ**. Which of this series of bones is most medial in position and which most lateral?

(d) There are small segments of bone present at **D**. Name these bones and state how they are maintained in this position in the live animal.

(e) Identify and name the pairs of bones which are marked **E**. In the live dog which structures are found lying in the space between the bone pairs?

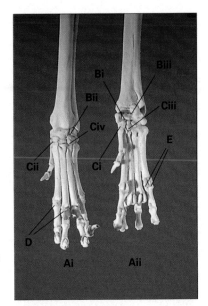

80. ▶

(a) Identify and name bone **Ai** and comment on the significance of the line marked **Aii** which appears to be running through it.

(b) Identify and name the bones which are marked **B**. Using criteria seen in this and the previous answer, state your reasons for identifying the species.

(c) Identify and name the bone which is outlined by the markers **C**.

(d) Identify and name bone **Di** and give the term for the prominence which is marked **Dii**.

(e) In the area of markers **E** there is a dark line giving the appearance of a deficiency in the tissue. What is the nature of the tissue found here and how can you explain this dark line?

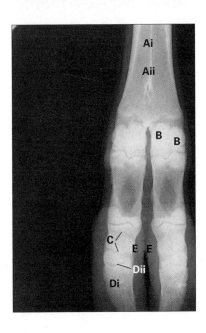

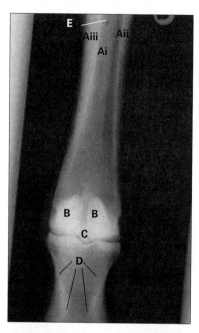

(a) Identify and name the individual bones marked **Ai**, **Aii** and **Aiii**. Which species is this?

(b) Identify and name the structures marked **B**. Which ligamentous connection lies between these structures and what anatomical landmark does it form here?

(c) The marker **C** is indicating a prominence. Name this prominence and state what region it lies in and its functional significance.

(d) The markers **D** are indicating a feature on the bony surface. What is producing this image and what attaches here in the live animal?

(e) Is this dark area, highlighted by marker **E**, a pathological or normal feature. Explain your answer.

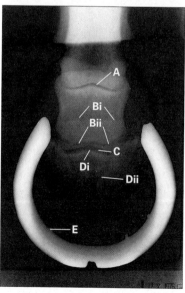

◀82.

(a) Identify and name the space marked **A**. State which bones lie around this space. Which species is this?

(b) Identify and name the outlined structure which lies between markers **Bi** and **Bii**. How is it maintained in this position in life?

(c) Identify and name the space which is marked **C** and state which types of movements are possible at this region.

(d) Identify and name the bone and the regions or features of that bone which are marked **Di** and **Dii**.

(e) What does the image marked **E** represent? Where should it be sited in relation to the structures lying immediately around it? State your reasons for identifying which foot is shown, fore or hind?

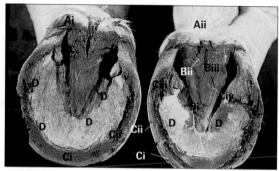

▲ 83.

(a) Identify and name the region, the aspect of this region and the species which is displayed here. Are the specimens **Ai** and **Aii** both from the same region of the animal? Give reasons for your answer.

(b) Identify and name structure **Bi** and the regions associated with that structure which are marked **Bii** and **Biii**.

(c) Give the terms which are applied to the regions marked **Ci**, **Cii**, **Ciii** and **Civ**.

(d) Give the regional name for the area marked **D** and identify what serves as the demarcation between regions **Ci** and **Cii** and the area marked **D**. What is the significance of this area of demarcation to the veterinarian?

(e) When contact is made with the ground surface, which of the previously identified structures would make initial impact and which would retain a weight-bearing contact with the ground?

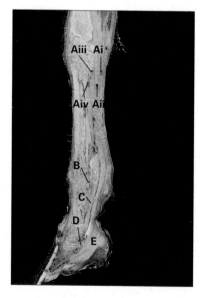

◀ 84.

(a) The coloured markers are indicating a series of structures which have been sectioned in long axis. Identify and name these structures marked thus: **Ai** (red), **Aii** (black), **Aiii** (blue) and **Aiv** (green).

(b) Identify and name the space which is marked **B**. Which bony structures lie around it?

(c) Identify and name the structure which attaches at **C**. What is it attaching to and which other structure, tendinous in nature, attaches here?

(d) Identify and name the structure which is marked **D** and state what lies on its dorsal and palmar surfaces.

(e) Identify and name the region which is marked **E**. What types of tissue are found here and what would be their function in the live animal? To which species would this animal belong?

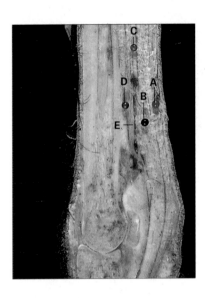

(a) The red marker **A** is inserted into
which structure? How does this
structure finally terminate?
(b) The black marker **B** is inserted into
which structure? How does this
structure finally terminate?
(c) The blue marker **C** is inserted into
which structure? How does this
structure finally terminate?
(d) The green marker **D** is inserted into
which structure? How does this
structure finally terminate?
(e) Identify and name the space marked **E**
and state the nature of its contents in
life.

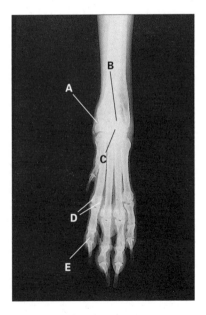

◀ 86.
(a) Identify and name prominence **A** and
name the bone it belongs to.
(b) Identify and name the whitened area
marked **B** and comment on the
intensity of the image.
(c) Identify and name the bone identified
by **C**.
(d) Identify and name the two bone
structures indicated by **D**. Describe
any structures which run between
them in life.
(e) Name the precise area marked **E** and
the bone on which it lies. What soft
tissue structure would be found
attached around here in life?

87. ▶

(a) Identify and name the vessel marked **A** and state which major vessel it arises from.

(b) Identify and name the vessel marked **B**.

(c) Identify and name the vessel marked **Ci** and also name the major branch marked **Cii**.

(d) Identify and name the vessel marked **Di** and the lesser vessel marked **Dii**.

(e) Identify and name the vessel marked **E** and state on which aspect of the limb it lies.

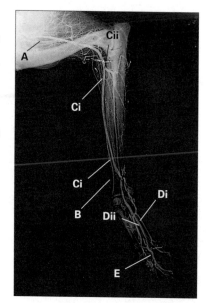

88. ▶

(a) Identify and name the vessel which is indicated by **A** and state which major vessel it finally flows into.

(b) Identify and name the vessel which is indicated by **B** and state which vessels it connects.

(c) Identify and name the vessel marked **C** and state which major vessel it flows into.

(d) Identify and name the vessel which is marked **D** and state which location in the body it is lying in.

(e) Of the vessels which have been identified so far, which would be used by the clinician for venepuncture and where in the body would this be performed?

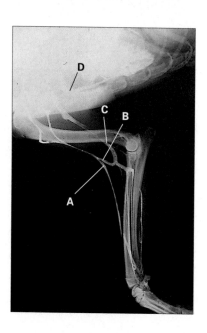

Thorax

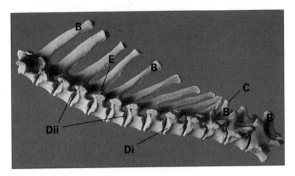

▲ 89.
(a) Identify and name this series of bones and indicate whether the most cranial bone of the series lies to the left or right.
(b) Identify and name the projections marked **B**. State what expansive extrinsic muscles of the thoracic limb originate from them and give details of the muscle insertions.
(c) Identify and precisely name bone **C** and discuss its number and significance in this series of bones.
(d) Identify and name areas **Di** and **Dii** and state what is found located in close approximation to these areas in life.
(e) Identify and name the small bony protuberance **E** and give the name of the bony projection it arises from.

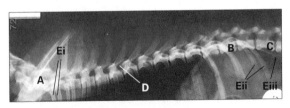

▲ 90.
(a) Identify precisely and name the individual bone marked **A**, stating where it is placed in the series of bones.
(b) Identify precisely and name the individual bone marked **B** and state where it is placed in the series of bones.
(c) Identify precisely and name the individual bone marked **C** and state where it is placed in the series of bones.
(d) Identify and name the aperture imaged at **D** and relate what structure would normally emerge here in life.
(e) Identify and name the individual bones marked **Ei**, **Eii** and **Eiii**. All of these bones articulate proximally with the vertebral column but how are they attached distally? Elaborate your answer for each of them.

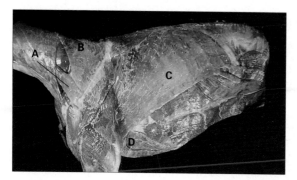

▲ 91.

(a) Identify and name muscle **A** and give a description of its origin, insertion and action.

(b) Identify and name muscle **B** and give a description of its origin, insertion and action.

(c) Identify and name muscle **C** and give an account of its origin, insertion and action.

(d) Identify and name muscle **D** and give an account of its origin, insertion and action.

(e) If the dog's brachial plexus had been completely torn would all or some of these muscles marked lose motor function? Explain your answer giving names.

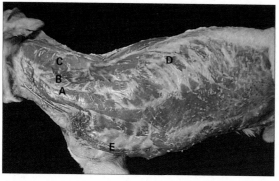

▲ 92.

(a) Identify and name muscle **A** and give its actions.

(b) Identify and name the muscle which has been cut at **B** in removal of the thoracic limb. Describe the origins and insertions of this muscle and state its actions.

(c) Identify and name muscle **C** and describe its actions.

(d) If a surgical incision were to be made through the intercostal space at position **D** name the layers of tissue which would be incised before access was gained into the thoracic cavity. If the incision were continued ventrally through the same intercostal space which muscle would be encountered?

(e) Identify and name the muscle group which has been cut at **E** to allow removal of the thoracic limb. State which bone this muscle group inserts on and indicate the motor nerve supply and the source of that nerve.

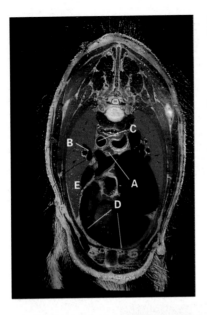

◀93.
(a) Identify and name the cross-sectioned organ marked **A**. Would this organ be seen in section at all levels through the length of the thorax or would it be missing at certain levels? Give details in your answer.

(b) Identify and name the cross-sectioned structure marked **B**. Describe the function of this structure and the nature of its wall.

(c) Identify and name the cross-sectioned organ marked **C**. Would this organ be seen in section at all levels through the length of the thorax or would it be missing at certain levels? Give details in your answer.

(d) Identify and name organ **D** and state what tissue layer surrounds it in the live animal.

(e) Identify and name the blood filled structure marked **E** and state which side of the body it lies, giving reasons for your answer.

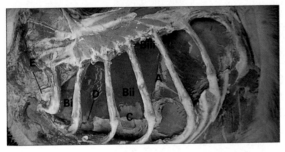

▲ 94.
(a) Identify and name the overall structure marked **A** and state which region is specifically indicated by the marker. What skeletal attachments does this structure make in the live dog?

(b) Identify and name the specific regions of this organ as they are marked **Bi**, **Bii** and **Biii**.

(c) Identify and name the organ, part of which can be seen at point **C**. Describe what layers of tissue overlie this organ as it is seen occupying its position at **C**.

(d) Identify and name the organ, part of which can be seen at point **D**. Is the presence of this organ in this position always present in every dog?

(e) The white area of tissue indicated at **E** represents a collective neurological structure. What is its name and what individual neurological elements run into it and where do they come?

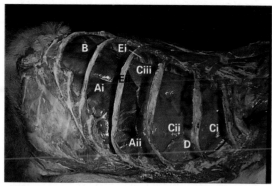

▲ 95.
(a) Identify and name the overall structure and the regions of it which are marked **Ai** and **Aii**. What is the function of this structure? Describe its nerve supply.
(b) Identify and name space **B** and state what forms its medial and lateral boundaries. What tissue layers cover the surfaces of these boundaries and what names do we apply to these layers?
(c) Identify and name the overall organ and the specific regions of it marked **Ci**, **Cii** and **Ciii**.
(d) Identify and name the space formed at **D** between structures **Ci** and **Cii**. What further structure can be seen placed at **D**?
(e) A collection of vascular and neurological structures are labelled **Ei** as they run through this area. Name these structures and describe their topographical relationship to structure **Eii** as they run along it. State the major connections that the vascular elements make with larger vessels of the region, giving names.

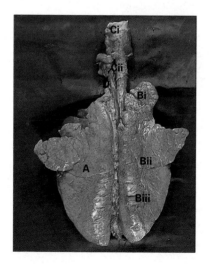

◀ 96.
(a) Identify and name the type of organ marked **A**.
(b) Identify and name the regions of this portion of the organ marked **Bi**, **Bii** and **Biii**.
(c) Identify and name the organs marked **Ci** and **Cii**.
(d) Identify and name the organ marked **D**.
(e) Using the criteria seen in the previous answers, identify the species giving your reasons.

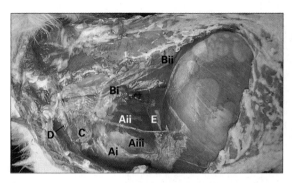

▲ 97.

(a) Identify and name the organ and the specific regions of it marked **Ai**, **Aii** and **Aiii**.
(b) Identify and name the structure labelled **Bi** and **Bii** and state where it originated and describe how and where it exits from the thoracic cavity.
(c) Identify and name organ **C** and give the topographical title of the intrathoracic position it occupies.
(d) Identify and name the vessels marked **D** and elaborate on the extent of the areas of the body which they supply.
(e) Identify and name precisely the section of an organ marked **E**. In life this is supported by a thin fold of tissue. Identify the type of tissue and name the fold, indicating the names of any other structures that are supported by it.

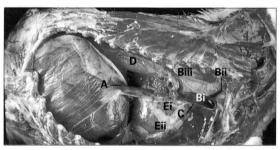

▲ 98.

(a) Identify and name area **A** and describe on which region of which structure it lies.
(b) Identify and name vessel **Bi** and state how it terminates caudally. Identify the contributing elements **Bii** and **Biii** and name the areas of the body which these contributories are responsible for.
(c) Identify and name the fine structure marked **C** and indicate how it originates and terminates.
(d) Identify and name the structure seen in region **D**, and name the fine strip of tissue which runs craniocaudally immediately under the marker. Explain how this fine structure enters and exits from the thorax.
(e) Identify and name the organ and the regions of it marked **Ei** and **Eii**. What name can be given to the region separating these two markers and what does it contain in life?

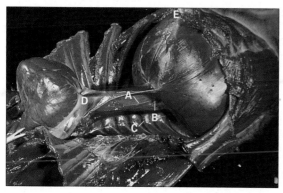

▲ 99.
(a) Identify and name the fine thread-like structure marked **A** and state on which organ it is lying. Describe how structure **A** passes between the abdominal and thoracic cavities, giving names.
(b) Identify and name vessel **B** and describe how it passes between the abdominal and thoracic cavities, giving names. Can you identify, with names, any other structure accompanying it at its point of passage?
(c) Identify and name the fine thread-like structure marked **C** and describe how it passes between the abdominal and thoracic cavities, giving names.
(d) Identify vessel **D** and describe how it passes between the abdominal and thoracic cavities, giving names.
(e) The marker **E** indicates a remnant of a bony structure which lay here in the midline in life. Name the segment of bone and identify of which larger bony structure it is part.

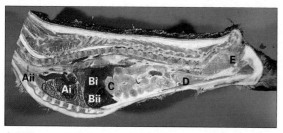

▲ 100.
(a) Name organ **Ai** and identify the structure which lies dorsal to it marked **Aii**. Why is **Aii** not evident caudal to this region?
(b) Identify and name organ **Bi** and state which structure is apparently seen within its substance marked **Bii**.
(c) Identify and name the organ, a portion of which is indicated by the marker **C**.
(d) Identify and name organ **D**. Is this the position that you would expect this organ to occupy at all times in the live dog?
(e) Identify and name organ **E** and name the bony structures which lie dorsal and ventral to it

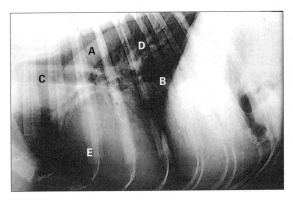

▲ **101.**

(a) Identify and name the structure imaged at **A** and state what points it runs between in the thorax.

(b) Identify and name the structure imaged at **B** and state what points it runs between in the thorax.

(c) Identify and name the structure imaged at **C** and state what points it runs between in the thorax.

(d) Identify and name the structures which can be seen imaged in area **D** and state which organ these structures are normally contained in.

(e) Identify and name the organ and the region of that organ which lies in area **E**.

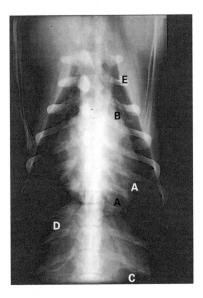

◀ **102.**

(a) Identify and name the organ and its topographical region marked **A**.

(b) Identify and name the organ and its topographical region marked **B**.

(c) Identify what the area imaged at **C** represents in the live animal.

(d) Identify and name the structures which are being imaged at the areas marked **D**.

(e) Does the marker **E** lie on the left or right side of the animal? Two of the previous answers can be used to validate your answer. Name them, with reasons.

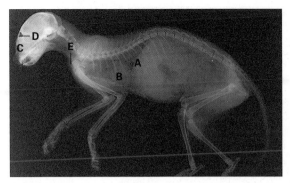

▲ 103.

(a) The marker placed at **A** is overlying a specific region which shows a narrow radio-opaque band apparently joining the concave contour of a larger structure. Interpret what is being imaged, giving specific names.

(b) If a one-and-a-half-inch needle were inserted through the region of marker **B** in this specific space in an entire animal, list in strict order what structures it might pass through. Where might its tip come to rest?

(c) Identify and name the bone of the skull marked **C**.

(d) Identify and name the bony region of the skull marked **D**.

(e) Identify and name the bony structure marked **E**. Does your answer assist you in naming this species? Give reasons, and state if any of the previous answers can further assist in species identification.

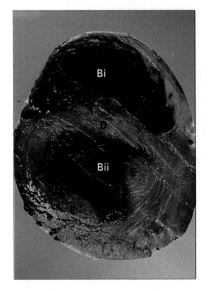

◀ 104.

(a) Identify and name the organ which has been sectioned here and state at which level the section has been made.

(b) Name the cavities which are marked **Bi** and **Bii** and identify one from the other giving reasons for your selection.

(c) In life would there be differences in the volume and the nature of the contents of these cavities?

(d) Identify and name the structure marked **D**.

(e) Identify and name the structures marked **E**. Name any structures that you know of which connect with **E** in life.

55

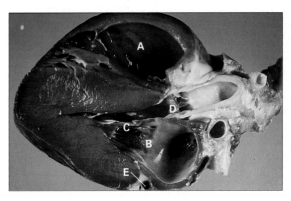

▲ 105.

(a) Identify and name the chamber marked **A** and give reasons for your selection. State the type of blood which would be flowing through here in life.

(b) Identify and name the structure marked **B** and describe its function and composition.

(c) Identify and name the elements marked **C**. To which structures do they attach and for what purpose?

(d) Identify structure **D** and state what it separates. Describe how it achieves this separation in life.

(e) Identify and name the structure sectioned at **E**. What nature of material would normally pass through this and where would it be travelling from and to in life?

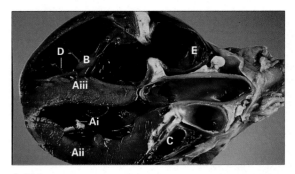

▲ 106.

(a) Identify and name chamber **Ai** and give reasons for your selection. Name the structures which form its boundaries at **Aii** and **Aiii**.

(b) Identify and name the structures marked **B**. State their function and attachments.

(c) Identify and name chamber **C**, and state the nature of the blood it contains in life.

(d) Identify and name structure **D** and state its course and points of attachment. What is its function and is a similar structure found in the chamber identified in **A**?

(e) Identify and name the type of structure occurring in the area marked **E**. What regions of the heart do you normally associate with this type of structure?

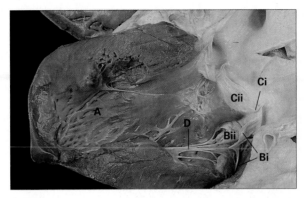

▲ **107.**

(a) Which region of which organ, marked **A**, has been opened here?

(b) Identify and name the type of structure marked **Bi** and state the term given to the region of it, marked **Bii**.

(c) Identify and name the type of structure marked **Ci** and state the term given to the region of it, marked **Cii**.

(d) Identify and name the structures marked **D**. What do they connect in the intact organ?

(e) Given the criteria seen in the previous answers identify which portion of the organ is shown and deduce specific names for structures **Bi** and **Ci**.

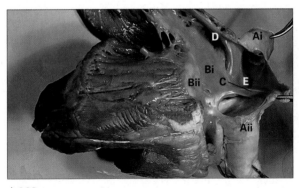

▲ **108.**

(a) Identify and name the vessels marked **Ai** and **Aii**.

(b) Identify and name the region of the organ marked **Bi** and state what structures **Bii** represents.

(c) Identify and name structure **C**.

(d) Identify and name the depressed region marked **D**.

(e) There is an area marked **E** where the covering surface has the appearance of a slit-like depression. What is this area called?

Abdomen and Pelvis

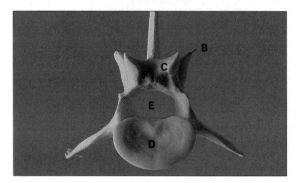

▲ **109.**

(a) Identify and name this type of bone and indicate what position it occupies in the sequence of bones of similar function, giving reasons for your selection.

(b) Identify and precisely name the area marked **B**.

(c) Identify and name the area marked **C** and state what relationship is formed by this and the next bone in the series.

(d) Identify and name the area marked **D** and state what relationship is formed by this and the next bone in the series.

(e) Identify and name aperture **E** and state what occupies this space in life. Include all relevant layers.

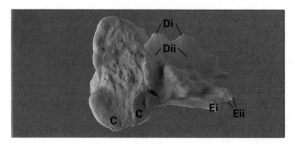

▲ **110.**

(a) Identify and name this bony object and state which aspect of it is shown. Where is it normally found in the live animal in relation to other bones of the series?

(b) What is the total bony composition of this structure as seen in the photograph?

(c) Identify and name area **C** and state on which region of the bony structure it is found. Which area of which other bony element does area **C** make a close approximation with in life? Describe the type of union formed including the function.

(d) Identify and name the prominences marked **Di** and **Dii**.

(e) Identify and name the areas marked **Ei** and **Eii** and state if any other bony structural surfaces are approximated to either of them in life.

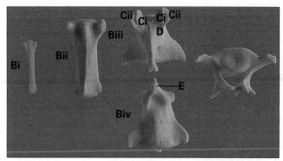

▲ 111.

(a) Identify and name the type of bones seen in this photograph and indicate where they would be situated in sequence in the entire animal.

(b) In this series of bones which of **Bi**, **Bii**, **Biii** and **Biv** would be the most cranial and which the most caudal? Give reasons for your selection.

(c) Identify and name the projections marked **Ci** and **Cii**. Do either or both of these articulate with another bone?

(d) Identify and name the plate of bone marked **D** and state what space within the bone it overlies. In life, what specific structures would be found passing through this space? Would you expect to find a similar space in all of the bones exhibited in this photograph? Give details of your opinion.

(e) Identify and name bony prominence **E** and state what space it overlies. What would pass through this space in the live animal?

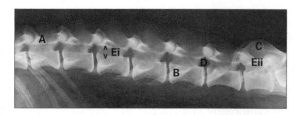

▲ 112.

(a) Identify and name bone **A** and state which number it is in this series of bones.

(b) Identify and name the structures marked **B** and name any muscles which might be found originating from them to run in a ventral direction.

(c) Identify and name bony area **C** and state which bone it is a part of.

(d) Identify and name the aperture which is imaged at area **D**. Name the neurological structure which emerges from this aperture in life and indicate what direction it runs in. Which area of the animal does the structure bear responsibility for?

(e) Identify and name the space which is imaged between the arrows at **Ei**. Explain what the contents of this space are in the live animal and comment on whether the contents would be identical in the same space at the level of **Eii**.

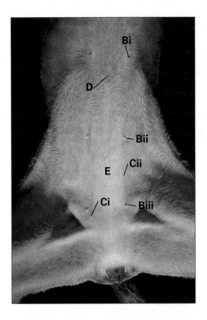

◀113.

(a) Name the species and sex of this animal giving one single major identifying feature seen on this exposure.

(b) Identify and name structures **Bi**, **Bii** and **Biii** and give a specific regional name for each of them.

(c) The marker **Ci** is indicating the region of a natural aperture, lying subcutaneously at this spot. A vessel, **Cii**, can be seen running cranially from this place. Name the aperture and the vessel.

(d) The marker is indicating a region of irregular skin at **D**. Name this area and state what it represents and describe what other structure might have been found here at a different period in this animal's life.

(e) The marker **E** is indicating a faint linear feature on the skin surface. Name this feature and describe what distinct linear region it would overlie in life.

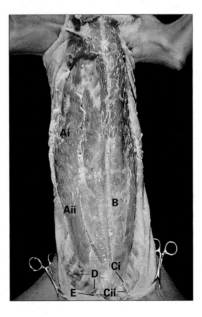

◀114.

(a) The markers **Ai** and **Aii** indicate a muscle of this region. Name the muscle and describe its origins and insertions.

(b) The marker **B** is lying on a fascial sheath which overlies a muscle. Name that muscle and describe its origins and insertions.

(c) The marker **Ci** indicates a natural aperture through which a collection of structures can be seen emerging at **Cii**. Name the aperture and describe its emerging contents.

(d) The area marked by the leader lines from **D** has a specific name and through it runs a number of vascular and neurological structures. Name the area and itemise the structures.

(e) The marker **E** indicates a small muscle belly. Name the muscle and give its function and motor nerve supply.

115. ▶

(a) The markers **Ai**, **Aii**, and **Aiii** are all indicating regions of one muscle. Name the overall muscle and give specific regional names to each marked portion which indicate the origins of these regions of the muscle.

(b) Identify the muscle indicated by marker **B** and describe its action and functional movements.

(c) The marker **C** is lying on a fascial sheet overlying a deeper muscle. Name that muscle and describe its origins.

(d) The marker **D** indicates a longitudinally running strand-like structure. Give this structure a specific name and discuss its relevance to the surgeon.

(e) Describe the relationships of the insertions of muscles **A**, **B** and **C** to the structure **D**.

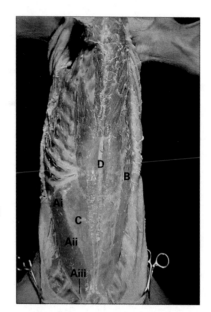

116. ▶

(a) Identify and name the prominent structure marked **A** and name the larger structure it forms a part of.

(b) Identify the structures which are marked at **B** and describe what they attach to.

(c) Identify and name the muscle which is marked at **Ci** and **Cii**. Which other muscle layers have been stripped off from these areas to reveal this muscle?

(d) Identify and name the structures which are indicated by the leader lines from **D**. What are they derived from? Be specific in your answer.

(e) Identify which muscle has been removed from area **E** and describe what deeper layers have been revealed by this action.

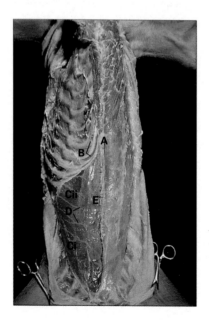

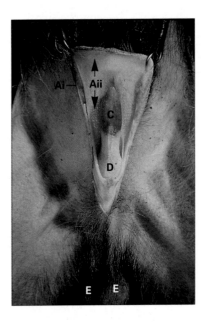

◀117.
(a) Identify and name the layer of tissue marked **Ai** and **Aii** and say which structure it forms a part of.
(b) The layer of tissue indicated in **Ai** contains fine strands of muscle. This can be seen in the folds of tissue on both sides. Name this muscle layer and state which muscle it is a segment of. What is the motor nerve supply to this muscle?
(c) Identify and name the organ and the region of the organ marked **C**.
(d) Identify and name the organ and the region of the organ marked **D**. What would be the source of arterial blood to region **D**?
(e) Identify and name the region marked **E**. What does this contain in life? If the contents were to be removed surgically, name in strict order the relevant layers of tissue which would be incised to expose and cut into the innermost contents.

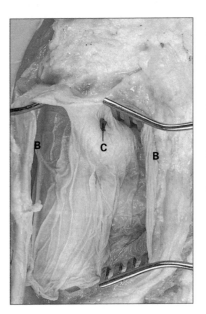

◀118.
(a) What structure is found in this region in a number of the domestic species?
(b) Upon opening into the named structure **B**, which organ would be found occupying the space found within it?
(c) In this case, a further space, marked **C**, seems to lead off from the original structure. What is this space termed and what is the species?
(d) What nature of material would normally be found filling space **C** in the live animal?
(e) What type of surface covering lines the area **B**?

119. ▶

(a) Identify and name aperture **A** and state what forms the boundaries of the opening both at this and deeper levels.

(b) Identify and name the composite structure marked **B** and list its total contents.

(c) Identify and name the organ which can be seen at **Ci** and state what layer of tissue is covering it at this level. Compare the appearance of this organ with that shown at **Cii**.

(d) Identify and name the muscle which is lying immediately to the left of marker **D**. What is its function and state which larger muscle it is part of.

(e) Identify and name the white tubular structure which can be seen running through area **E**. Where precisely does it originate from and what is its final destination?

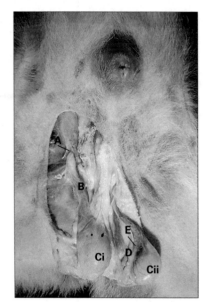

120. ▶

(a) Identify and name the aperture marked **A**.

(b) The aperture occurs in a sheet of tissue marked **B**. What does this layer represent and what is it called?

(c) Identify and name the muscle marked **C** and state its regions of origin and insertion. What type of muscle is it?

(d) Which structure is muscle **C** overlying?

(e) A similar opening lies at position **E**. Which part of which organ lies covered by connective tissue in the space between **A** and **E**?

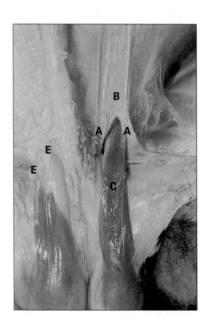

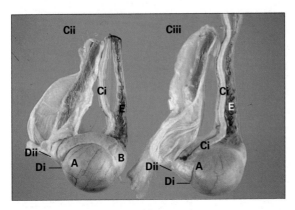

▲ 121.
(a) Identify and name the organ and the region of the organ marked **A**.
(b) Identify and name the structure and the region of the structure marked **B**.
(c) Identify and name the structure marked **Ci**. Indicate which marker, **Cii** or **Ciii** signifies the lateral aspect of the organ shown. Give reasons for your answer.
(d) Identify and name the connecting areas of tissue marked **Di** and **Dii**. During the processes of open and closed castration which of these must be severed to remove the testis?
(e) Identify and name the vessels and the nature of their configuration as they are marked at **E**. Describe the functional significance of this arrangement.

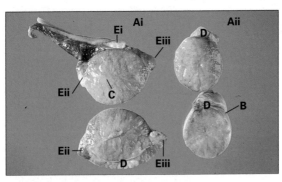

▲ 122.
(a) Identify and name the organ shown and describe the planes of section of **Ai** and **Aii**.
(b) Identify and name the outer layers marked **B**.
(c) Identify and name the region of the organ marked **C**. What minute structures run through this area?
(d) Name the structure and region of this structure marked **D**. What type of physiological process is ongoing in this region?
(e) Which structure does marker **Ei** point to? Does this structure commence at extremity **Eii** or extremity **Eiii**?

123. ▶

(a) Identify and name the organ marked **A**.

(b) Identify and name the structure and the region of that structure marked **B**. Can you explain the colouration and, giving suitable anatomical reasons, can you identify the species?

(c) Identify and name the structure and the region of that structure marked **C** and give details of any structures which you know of which may be entering or leaving region **C**. Describe the topographical positioning of **C** in relation to other landmarks in the live animal

(d) Identify and name the fold of tissue marked **D**, giving an explanation of the position it occupies in real life.

(e) Identify the muscle marked **E**, stating what type of muscle tissue it contains and from where it takes origin.

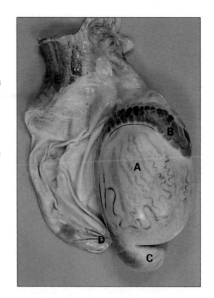

124. ▶

(a) Identify and name the organ marked **A** and describe the plane in which it has been sectioned.

(b) Identify and name the outermost layers which are marked **B** and describe the nature of the tissues involved.

(c) Identify and name the layers of tissue which are marked **C**. Describe the nature of the tissue and the cell types which constitute the areas between the lines of tissue marked **C**.

(d) Identify and name the region of the organ which is marked **D**. What type of tissues make up the infrastructure of this region?

(e) From the region marked **D**, describe the method and direction of movement of the products of the organ **A**.

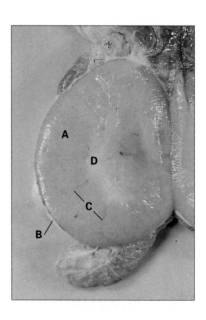

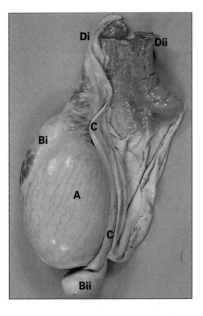

◀ 125.

(a) Identify and name the type of organ marked **A**, and state in sequence which layers of tissue have been cut through, starting at the skin surface, to reveal this aspect of the organ.

(b) Identify and name the structure and the regions of that structure which are marked **Bi** and **Bii**.

(c) Identify and name the tubular structure marked **C** and state its eventual proximal destination.

(d) If an incision were made totally across the structures between markers **Di** and **Dii**, name all the vascular elements from which one could anticipate haemorrhage.

(e) Using the information gained from observing the external appearance of the organ and related structures, identify the species. State the topographical position which the structures found in the region marked **Di** and **Dii** would occupy normally. Relate them to any other external organs of the same body system of the animal.

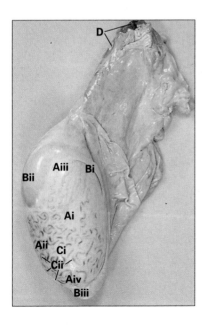

◀ 126.

(a) Identify the type of organ seen here marked **Ai** and name the regions of it which are indicated **Aii**, **Aiii** and **Aiv**.

(b) Name the structure which is marked **Bi** and identify the regions of it which are marked **Bii** and **Biii**.

(c) Identify and name the covering surfaces over which the marker **Ci** is lying and name the structures which can be seen beneath them as indicated by the markers **Cii**.

(d) Identify and name the structure which is marked **D** and state what its function is in life.

(e) Using the criteria seen in the previous answers, state your reasons for identifying this species.

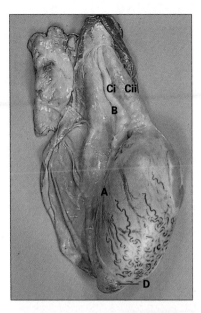

◀ 127.
(a) Identify and name the type of organ and the region of that organ which is displayed here marked **A**.
(b) Identify and name the structure which is marked **B**. State its function and the connections it makes proximally and distally.
(c) Identify and name the composite structure which is lying between the markers **Ci** and **Cii**. Through the outer covering it is possible to see vascular structures arranged in a particular manner. Describe this arrangement giving a name and its function.
(d) Identify and name the connection which is being made between the adjacent organs at **D**.
(e) Using the criteria seen in the previous answers name, giving reasons, the species and the aspect of the organ displayed here.

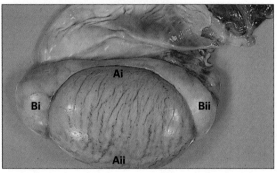

128. ▲
(a) Identify the type of organ which is displayed here and name the regions of it which are marked **Ai** and **Aii**.
(b) Identify and name the structure and the regions of that structure which are marked **Bi** and **Bii**.
(c) Using the visual evidence which is evident in the photograph, identify the species, giving your reasons.
(d) Given the species you have identified, state the topographical position that you would expect this organ to occupy in the live animal.
(e) In this particular species, orientate the structures which are marked **Bi** and **Bii** in relation to the direction they occupy in the body.

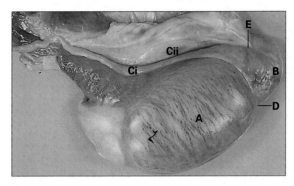

▲ 129.

(a) Identify and name the type of organ displayed here at **A**.
(b) Identify and name the structure and region of that structure marked **B**.
(c) Identify and name the structure marked **Ci** and describe its function. What specific term is given to the fold of tissue marked **Cii** which lies adjacent to the structure **Ci**.
(d) Identify and name the connecting strand of tissue marked **D**.
(e) Identify and name the connecting strand of tissue marked **E**.

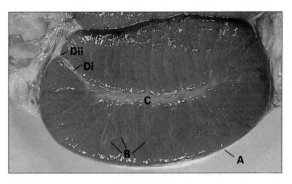

▲ 130.

(a) Identify and name this type of organ and give the term for its outer layer of tissue marked **A**.
(b) Give the name applied to the strands of tissue which are marked **B** and describe the nature of the tissue which lies between these strands naming any specific cell types which are found there.
(c) Identify and name the region of the organ which is marked **C**. Which tubular system does it contain?
(d) Identify and name the contents of the strand of tissue which is marked **Di** and state to which area it leads at **Dii**.
(e) Using the criteria which has been seen in the previous answers, name the species giving reasons for your choice.

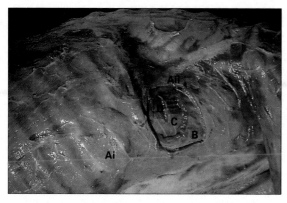

▲ 131.

(a) Identify and name muscle layer **Ai** and **Aii**. Give your reason for identifying and naming this layer compared with the other layers shown in this dissection.

(b) Identify and name muscle layer **B** which appears through the aperture in the dissection. Give a reason for your decision compared with the other layers.

(c) Identify and name muscle layer **C** which appears through the aperture in the dissection. Give a reason for your decision compared with the other layers.

(d) If an incision were continued through layer **C** what other layers of tissue would be encountered? Where would the surgeon's interrogating instrument now be located?

(e) If a pair of forceps were carefully introduced through incision **D** what organs might be encountered and grasped at this specific area?

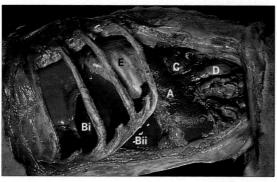

▲ 132.

(a) Identify and name the organ marked **A**.

(b) Identify and name the organ marked **Bi** and **Bii**, giving the regional names of these two marked areas.

(c) Identify and name the organ marked **C**.

(d Identify and name the organ and the portion of that organ marked **D**.

(e) Identify and name the organ marked **E** and state what area of that organ the marker overlies.

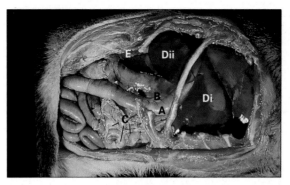

▲ 133. This is the lateral aspect of the thoracic and abdominal regions of a dog after removal of the overlying musculature and some ribs. The diaphragm has also been partially removed.

(a) Identify and name the organ and the region of the organ marked **A**.

(b) Identify and name organ **B** which is lying immediately adjacent to organ **A**.

(c) Identify and name the organ and the region of the organ indicated by the markers **C**. State what layers of tissue can be seen overlying these portions of the organ.

(d) Identify and name the organ and the regions of the organ marked **Di** and **Dii**.

(e) Identify and name organ **E**. Give a name to the portion of organ **D** which lies immediately cranioventral to it.

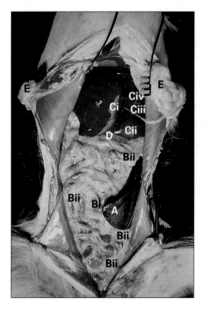

◄ 134. This is the ventral aspect of an abdominal region of a male dog after resection of the abdominal musculature.

(a) Identify and name organ **A** and identify which extremity of the organ this is.

(b) Identify and name the structures which can be seen in the region marked **Bi** and name the overlying layers of tissue which can be seen in a superficial position marked **Bii**.

(c) Identify and name the organ and the regions of the organ marked **Ci**, **Cii**, **Ciii** and **Civ**.

(d) Identify and name the organ and the limited portion of the organ marked **D** which can be seen extending beyond the edge of organ **Cii**.

(e) Identify and name the layer of tissue marked **E** and discuss its points of attachment in the intact abdomen.

135. ▶

(a) Identify and name the fold of fat-laden tissue marked **A** which has been reflected to lie in this lateral position. State which organs this fold attaches to and comment on whether the fold of tissue has been sectioned in any way to accomplish this reflection.

(b) Identify and name the portion of intestine which is indicated by the markers **B**.

(c) Identify and name the portion of intestine marked **C**, and describe which direction it is travelling in within the abdominal cavity.

(d) Identify and name organ **Di** and also name the fold of tissue attaching to it marked **Dii**.

(e) Identify and name the structure which is seen at the position marked **E** and name the organ lying immediately caudal to it. State how this organ attaches to structure **E** in life.

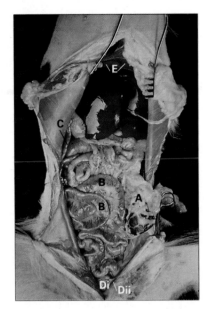

136. ▶

(a) Identify and name the portion of intestine marked **A** and state in which direction it is travelling in the abdomen.

(b) Identify and name organ **B** and state in which fold of tissue it lies.

(c) Identify and name the portions of intestine marked **Ci** and **Cii** and state the source of arterial blood to this region of the intestine.

(d) Identify and name the portion of intestine marked **D** and state to where and by which route its venous drainage flows.

(e) Identify and name the fold of tissue over which marker **E** is lying. Identify all types of vessels which might be flowing through this fold giving the destination of each type of vessel.

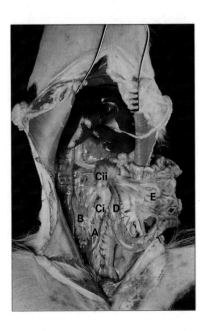

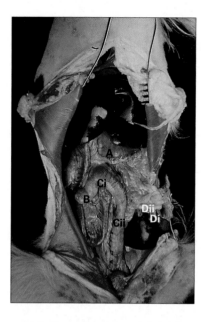

◀ **137.** Portions of the intestine have been resected.

(a) Identify and name the organ and the area of that organ marked **A**. What would be the source of arterial blood to this region of the organ?

(b) What organs have been removed by sectioning the intestine at the level marked **B**?

(c) Name the organ and the regions of the organ marked **Ci** and **Cii** and the name of the fold of tissue which supports them.

(d) Identify and name the organ marked **Di** and state the name of the fold of tissue which is seen related to it at **Dii**.

(e) Which source is the arterial flow to organ **D** derived from and to where and by which route would the venous blood be travelling from organ **D**?

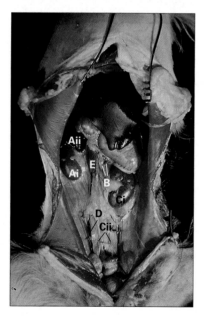

◀ **138.** The entire intestinal tract has been removed from this male dog.

(a) Identify and name organ **Ai** and the region of the organ which is lying immediately cranial to it at **Aii**.

(b) Identify and name the small whitish organs which are indicated by the markers **B**. What is the name of the vessels which can be seen running across the area between these organs?

(c) Identify and name organ **Ci** and name the tubular structures which are indicated by the markers **Cii**. Where are structures **Cii** running from and to as they lie in the abdominal cavity?

(d) Identify and name the structures marked **D** and state where they are running from and to as they lie in the abdominal cavity.

(e) Identify and name the vessel which is indicated by marker **E**. Where is this vessel running to? At this particular point in its course, would the blood it contains be related to organs **Aii** and **Ci**?

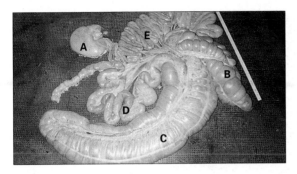

▲ 139.
(a) Identify and name the organ marked **A**.
(b) Identify and name the organ marked **B**.
(c) Identify and name the organ marked **C**.
(d) Identify and name the organ marked **D**.
(e) Identify and name the organ marked **E** and using the criteria gained from the previous answers name the species shown here.

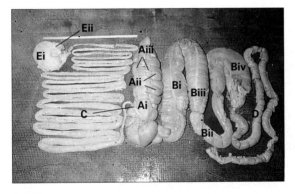

▲ 140.
(a) Identify and name the organ marked **Ai** and give the species. State also the name and composition of the specific structures marked **Aii** and **Aiii**.
(b) Identify and name the organ marked **Bi** and state the name of the precise areas of that organ which are marked **Bii**, **Biii** and **Biv**.
(c) Identify and name the tubular structure which is marked **C** and state how it is related to structure **Ai**.
(d) Identify and name the structure marked **D** and describe the nature and appearance of its contents in life.
(e) Identify and name the organ **Ei** and the specific region of that organ marked **Eii**.

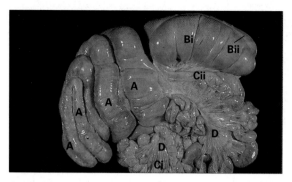

▲ **141.** This set of viscera has been removed from the abdominal cavity.

(a) Identify and name the organ which is marked **A** and state the nature of its spatial configuration.

(b) Identify and name the organ marked **Bi** and state what type of structure is indicated by the marker **Bii**.

(c) Identify and precisely name the tubular structures marked **Ci** and **Cii**.

(d) Identify and name the layer of tissue marked **D** and describe the nature of the structures which can be seen running through it. What would be the origins and destinations of these structures?

(e) Using the criteria seen in the previous answers, identify this species.

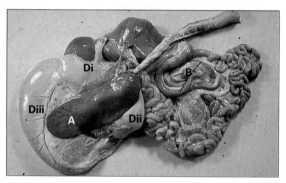

▲ **142.** This is a set of viscera removed from an abdominal cavity.

(a) Identify and name the organ which is marked **A**.

(b) Identify and name the structures which are indicated by the markers **B**.

(c) Using the criteria gained from the answers for **A** and **B**, name the species which is demonstrated here.

(d) Identify and name the organs marked **Di**, **Dii** and **Diii** giving topographical landmarks to support your decisions.

(e) Using the information gained from the answers in (d) can you give an opinion of the degree of maturity of the individual animal to which these organs belonged? Give reasons for your answer.

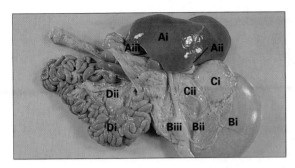

▲ **143.**

(a) Identify and name the organ marked **Ai** and name the areas of that organ which are marked **Aii** and **Aiii**.

(b) Identify and name the organ which is marked **Bi** and name the regions of that organ which are marked **Bii** and **Biii**.

(c) Identify and name the organ which is marked **Ci** and state the name and nature of the tissue of the fold marked **Cii**.

(d) Identify and name the organs which are marked **Di** and name the fold of tissue marked **Dii** plus the vessels which are to be seen running in it. What would be their parent vessels?

(e) With the information detected in the answers (a), (b) and (c), identify, giving reasons, the species and age group of the animal from which these viscera were taken.

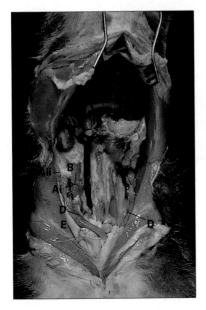

◀ **144.** This is a cat from which the entire intestinal tract has been removed.

(a) Identify and name organ **Ai** and state the name of the strand of tissue which is seen running cranially from it and marked **Aii**.

(b) Identify the vessels marked **B** and describe their origins and areas of responsibility.

(c) If organ **Ai** were to be removed surgically would ligaturing vessels **B** be sufficient to allow a haemorrhage-free resection? Give reasons.

(d) Identify and name the organ and region of that organ marked **D** and state the name of the fold of tissue supporting it.

(e) Identify and name the natural aperture which is apparent in area **E** and describe the structures in which it forms an aperture. State the name of the tissue fold which appears to pass into this area of the aperture.

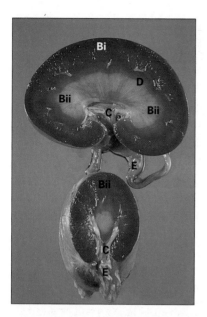

◀ 145.

(a) Identify the organ displayed and give the species, eliminating other species with which it might be confused.

(b) Identify and name the areas **Bi** and **Bii**, explaining the reasons for the distinct difference in texture and colour.

(c) Identify and name the region of the organ marked **C** and state what material is found in this region in life.

(d) Identify and name the vessels indicated by the markers **D** and describe their subsequent ramifications, giving names.

(e) Identify and name the tubular structure marked **E** and state its region of origin and its final destination.

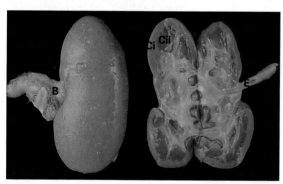

▲ 146.

(a) Identify these organs and, using a description based only on information from the intact organ, state which species they belong to.

(b) Identify and name the region of the organ marked **B** and state which structures course through this area in life.

(c) Identify and name the regions of the sectioned organ which are marked **Ci** and **Cii**.

(d) Using only information derived from the sectioned organ, confirm your original answer for species of organ.

(e) Identify and name the structure which has been opened into at **E** and state what it connects with in life, briefly describing its course through the body.

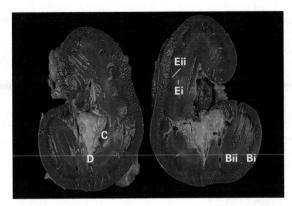

▲ 147.
(a) Identify the organs which have been sectioned and name the species, giving reasons for your selection.
(b) Identify and name the regions of the organs which are marked **Bi** and **Bii**.
(c) Identify and name the region of the organ marked **C**.
(d) Identify and name the region of the organ marked **D** and state whether this arrangement is found in the other domesticated species.
(e) Identify and name the vessels which are marked **Ei** and **Eii**.

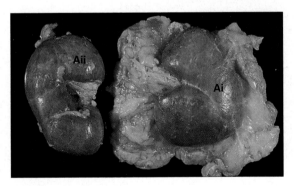

▲ 148.
(a) Identify and name the type of organs displayed in this photograph as **Ai** and **Aii**.
(b) Name the species to which they belong giving reasons concerning their external appearance to justify your answer.
(c) Identify between **Ai** and **Aii** as to which is the left and which is the right-sided organ.
(d) Giving a suitable topographical description, indicate where in the body these structures are normally found.
(e) Name two types of endocrine organs which lie in close proximity to these organs in the live animal.

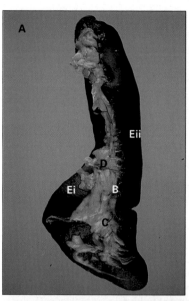

◀ 149.

(a) Identify and name the organ displayed here, giving the species, and state which aspect of it is displayed in **A**.

(b) Identify and name the region of the organ indicated by the markers **B**.

(c) Identify and name the fold of tissue which is indicated by the marker **C**. Which larger structure is it a part of?

(d) Identify and name the vessels which are indicated at **D** and state where they are running from and going to.

(e) Describe which organs might lie against the surfaces marked **Ei** and **Eii** in the living animal.

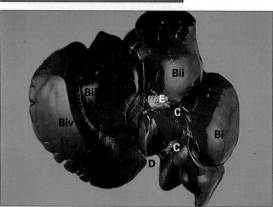

▲ 150.

(a) Identify and name this organ. Give the species and describe which aspect of the organ is being viewed.

(b) Identify and name the regions of the organ marked **Bi**, **Bii**, **Biii** and **Biv**.

(c) Identify and name the vessel marked **C**. Is it carrying blood from or to the major organ and which routes are used in the process?

(d) State at which border of the organ the marker **D** is situated.

(e) Identify and name the fragment of tissue which is marked **E** and state which structures attach it to the major organ in the live animal.

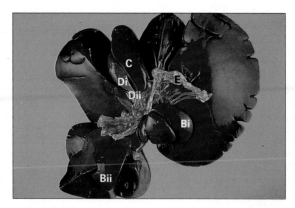

▲ 151.
(a) Identify this organ and describe the aspect of the organ that is being viewed.
(b) Identify and name the areas of the organ marked **Bi** and **Bii**.
(c) Identify and name the area of the organ marked **C** and state which border of the major organ the free edge of this area reaches to.
(d) Identify and name the structure marked **Di** and indicate the name of its continuation which is marked **Dii**. What are the functions of these structures?
(e) Identify and name the fold of tissue which is marked **E** and name any organs and the regions of these organs to which it attaches.

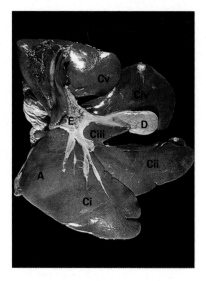

◄ 152.
(a) Identify this organ and name the species, giving two major criteria for your selection of species.
(b) Describe and name the surface of the organ.
(c) Name the regions of the organ which are marked **Ci**, **Cii**, **Ciii**, **Civ** and **Cv**.
(d) Identify and name the structure marked **D**. What type of material does it contain in the live animal and by what means does this material enter and leave the structure.
(e) Identify and name the region marked **E** and name all the structures which pass through this region.

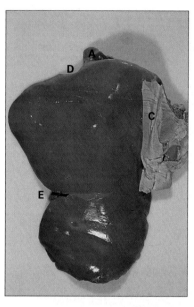

◀ 153.

(a) Identify the organ and the portion of the organ marked **A** and suggest the possible species type, giving reasons for your selection.

(b) Identify which aspect of this organ is shown and state in which direction this aspect would be directed in the live animal.

(c) Identify and name the sectioned structure marked **C** and state which part of the entire structure this represents.

(d) Identify and name the border of the organ and the indentation on that border marked **D** and state what lies in close relationship with this indentation in life.

(e) Identify and name the indentation in the border of the organ marked **E** and state whether this lies to the left or right of midline in life.

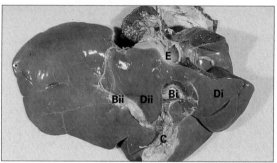

▲ 154.

(a) Identify and name the type of organ displayed here and give an indication of the type of species from which it comes, giving reasons.

(b) By identifying the structures marked **Bi** and **Bii**, name which aspect of the organ is displayed here.

(c) At region **C** the trimmed edges of a structure which has been largely removed can be seen. What would have been present here in life and on which side of the animal's body would it have been found?

(d) Identify and name the regions of the organ which are marked **Di** and **Dii**.

(e) Identify and name the structure which has been sectioned at **E** and comment on the reason for the apparent perforations which can be seen on its interior surface. Where would structure **E** lie in the live animal?

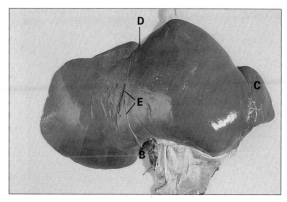

▲ 155.

(a) Identify and name the type of organ displayed here and give reasons for selecting a species type.

(b) Identify and name which aspect of the organ is displayed here and state whether the marked area **B** indicates the left or right margin of the organ.

(c) Identify and name the region of the organ marked **C** and comment on whether this would further support your selection of species type.

(d) Identify and name the indentation marked **D** and comment on what could occupy this space in life.

(e) Identify and name the structure which is seen on the surface of the organ at **E**.

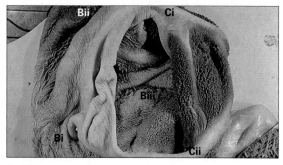

▲ 156.

(a) Identify the opened organ and name the possible species, giving reasons.

(b) By identifying and describing the nature of the surface coverings of the regions marked **Bi** and **Bii** state which part of the organ the opening incision been made into? Therefore, which region of the organ are we looking into at **Biii**?

(c) Name the regions marked **Ci** and **Cii** and explain their physical appearance compared with the surrounding areas.

(d) What is the source of innervation for this organ and how would the nerve/nerves involved reach the organ?

(e) Name the major the blood supply to and from this organ and state the origins and destinations of the vessels involved.

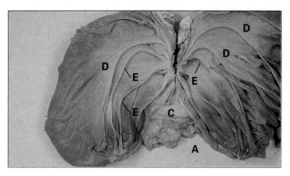

▲ 157.
(a) This organ has been been incised to reveal the interior of a chamber. Identify and name the organ and give the possible species from which it has been removed.
(b) This chamber is one in a sequence of chambers. Indicate its numerical position in this sequence.
(c) The marker **C** is indicating a specific region of the organ. Name this region and indicate what its functional significance is and what it interconnects.
(d) Identify the structures which are marked **D** and describe their surface covering.
(e) There are spaces between the structures **D** which are indicated by the pointers **E**. Give the name for these spaces. If the spaces were revealed by separating the structures **C** what would be found there in life?

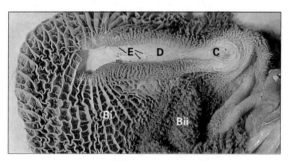

▲ 158.
(a) An incision has been made into some of the abdominal viscera. Name which group of organs have been incised and suggest from which possible species they have been removed.
(b) By describing the surfaces marked at **Bi** and **Bii**, positively identify which individual organs are involved.
(c) Identify, with reasons, the region marked **C** and describe what actions occur here in life and under which circumstances.
(d) Identify, with reasons, the region marked **D** and describe what actions take place here in life and under which circumstances?
(e) The markers **E** are indicating precise raised structures on the surface of region **D**. Name these structures.

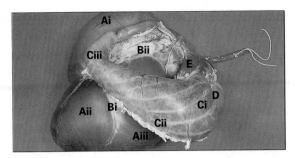

▲ **159.**
(a) Identify and name the organ and the regions of that organ marked **Ai**, **Aii** and **Aiii**.
(b) Name the regions of the organ which are marked **Bi** and **Bii**.
(c) Identify and name the organ and the regions of that organ marked **Ci**, **Cii** and **Ciii**.
(d) Identify and name the organ marked **D** and name the structures which it lies in close apposition with in the live animal.
(e) Identify and name the organ marked **E**. Which of the organs **A**, **B** and **C** does it directly communicate with?

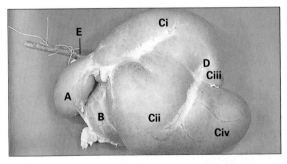

▲ **160.**
(a) Identify and name the organ marked **A** and state what other structures it would lie in close association with in life.
(b) Identify and name the organ marked **B** and describe where it would normally be situated in the live animal.
(c) Identify and name the organ and the regions of that organ which are marked **Ci**, **Cii**, **Ciii** and **Civ**. Which aspect of the organ are we looking at?
(d) Identify and name the marked furrow which is indicated at **D** and state what structures might be found occupying this furrow in life. Give the origins or destinations of the structures.
(e) Identify and name the organ which is marked **E**. What type of tissue forms its wall and what would be the possible sources of blood flow to the wall of this organ at region **E**?

83

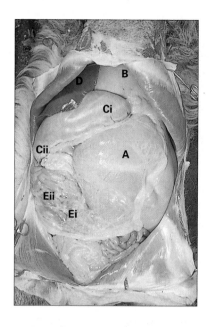

◀ **161.** This specimen demonstrates the
   ventral aspect of an open abdominal
   cavity of a sheep.
(a) Identify and name the organ marked **A**.
(b) Identify and name the organ marked
   B.
(c) Identify and name the organ and the
   regions of that organ marked **Ci** and
   Cii.
(d) Identify and name the organ marked **D**.
(e) Identify and name the membranous
   structure which can be seen marked
   Ei and state what structures, **Eii**, are
   visible lying deep to this membrane.
   What specific name can be given to
   this space where these structures
   labelled **Eii** are lying?

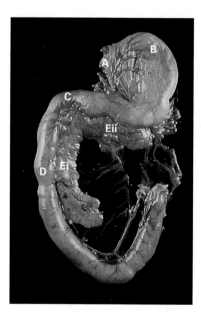

◀ **162.**
(a) Giving species, identify and name the
   organ and the region of the organ
   marked **A**. Where would this be found
   in the live animal and what has been
   sectioned to allow removal of this
   organ from the body cavity?
(b) Identify and name the region of the
   organ marked **B** and state where this
   lies in the intact animal. Comment on
   whether this is in a constant position
   at all times in the live animal.
(c) Identify and name the region of the
   organ marked **C** and state where this
   would lie in the intact animal.
(d) Identify and name the organ and the
   region of that organ marked **D** and
   state where it lies in the intact animal.
(e) Identify and name the organ and the
   regions of that organ which are
   marked **Ei** and **Eii**. Name the function
   of this organ and describe how it is
   related to structures **C** and **D**.

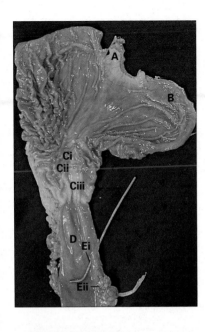

◀ **163.** This organ has been removed from the abdominal cavity and opened to reveal its interior.

(a) Identify and name the organ and indicate the region and the type of glandular elements which are found in the region marked **A**.

(b) Identify and name the region of the organ marked **B** and indicate the type of glandular elements which are found here.

(c) Identify and name the region of the organ marked **Ci**, **Cii** and **Ciii** and indicate the type of glandular elements which are found in these areas.

(d) Identify the organ which has been opened here and describe the nature of the surface covering of the area marked **D**.

(e) Identify and name the orifices which are indicated by markers **Ei** (probe in opening) and **Eii**. State what opens through these apertures in the live animal.

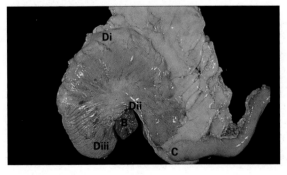

▲ **164.**

(a) Identify and name the type of organ displayed here.

(b) Identify and name the structure which is marked **B** and name the region where it is situated, relative to the major organ.

(c) Identify and name the structure which is marked **C** and name the region where it is situated, relative to the major organ.

(d) Identify and name the regions of the organ which are marked **Di**, **Dii** and **Diii**.

(e) Using criteria given in your previous answers and any other clues present surrounding the organ, identify this species giving reasons for your choice.

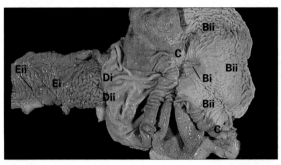

▲ **165.** This organ has been sectioned and arranged to display its interior lining.

(a) Identify and name this type of organ.

(b) Identify and name the aperture which is marked **Bi** and give the name of the region which surrounds it, marked **Bii**.

(c) Identify and name the distinct line effect which the marker **C** is overlying. Using the criteria which you have given in this and the previous answers, name, giving reasons, this species.

(d) Identify and name the region of the organ which is marked **Di** and state what the raised area, which the marker **Dii** overlies, is representing.

(e) Identify and name the organ which is marked **Ei**. The marker **Eii** is pointing to a raised structure on the surface of the organ. What is this called and what is its functional significance?

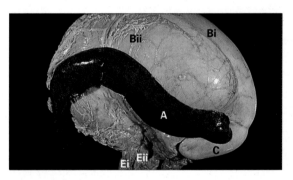

▲ **166.**

(a) Identify and name the type of organ marked **A** and state what surface of that organ is displayed here.

(b) Identify and name the type of organ marked **Bi** and state the nature and name of the layer of tissue which is seen overlying the organ at **Bii**.

(c) Identify and name the region of organ **B** which bears the marker **C**.

(d) Using the criteria which has been given in the previous answers, identify this species giving reasons for your choice.

(e) Identify and name the organs which are marked **Ei** and **Eii**.

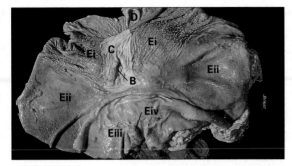

▲ 167. This organ has been sectioned to display its interior lining.
(a) Identify and name the type of organ which is displayed here.
(b) Identify and name the opening which is indicated by the marker **B** and state what enters here.
(c) Identify and name the region of the organ which is marked **C** and describe the nature of its surface covering.
(d) Identify and name the region of the organ which is marked **D** and, using the criteria from this and the previous answers, identify this species, giving reasons for your answer.
(e) Identify and name the regions of the organ which are marked **Ei**, **Eii** and **Eiii**, commenting on the nature of the lining. In region **Eiii** there is an elevated portion marked **Eiv**. Name this elevation and comment on the functional significance of its position.

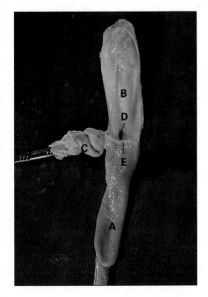

◄ 168. This represents the point of junction of the small with the large intestine. The tubular tract has been opened to reveal the interior.
(a) Identify the region of the tubular tract marked **A** and give two major factors regarding its appearance which support your answer.
(b) Identify the region of the tubular tract marked **B** and give two major factors regarding its appearance which support your answer.
(c) Identify and name the portion of the tubular tract marked **C**. State, with reasons, which species it belongs to.
(d) Identify and name the aperture marked **D** indicating what it connects.
(e) The raised ridge of tissue marked **E** would represent what structure and which opening in the live animal?

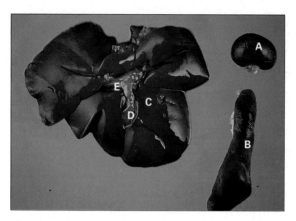

▲ 169.

(a) Identify and name organ **A** and name the species, giving reasons.
(b) Identify and name organ **B** and state which surface of the organ is shown.
(c) Identify and name organ **C** and state which surface of the organ shown.
(d) Identify and name structure **D** and state which portions of **C** lie to the left and right of it.
(e) Identify and name the region of organ **C** which is indicated by the marker **E**. List all the structures which might be found passing to and from the organ at this area.

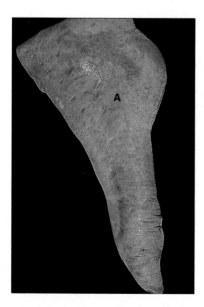

◀ 170.

(a) Identify and name the type of organ marked **A**.
(b) Identify which aspect of the organ is shown.
(c) Identify this species, giving reasons for your selection.
(d) In life, which other organ is **A** most closely related to?
(e) Using bony landmarks, describe where organ **A** would lie in the live animal.

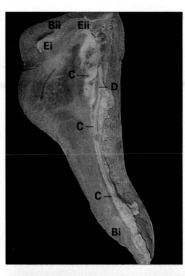

◄171.

(a) Identify this type of organ and state which aspect is shown.

(b) State the direction in which markers **Bi** and **Bii** orientate when this organ is lying in the animal's body.

(c) Identify and name the region of the organ indicated by **C** and describe what structure can be found attaching along this area. Using the criteria which has been given so far, identify the species giving reasons for your choice.

(d) Identify and name vessel **D** and state its major vessel of origin.

(e) Identify and name the structures which are seen arising from the regions marked **Ei** and **Eii** and state which other organs or structures they attach to.

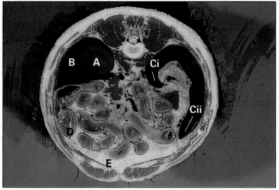

▲ 172. This is the cranial face of a transverse section through the abdominal region of a dog.

(a) Identify and name organ **A** and give a reason for the two distinct colour layers shown on this cross-section.

(b) Identify and name the organ and the region of the organ marked **B**. Is this the left or right side of the animal? Give reasons for your answer.

(c) Identify and name organ **Ci** and **Cii**. Indicte the regions of the organ which the markers point to.

(d) Identify and name organ **D**, giving a precise identification of the portion of the organ which has been cut in cross-section.

(e) Identify and name tissue fold **E** and state which muscles it is lying immediately dorsal to in this section.

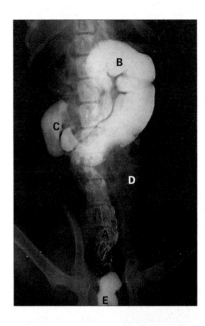

173. This is a ventrodorsal radiograph of the abdomen of a dog to which a barium enema has been administered.

(a) Identify and name the portion of the intestinal tract which is imaged at **A**.

(b) Identify and name the portion of the intestinal tract which is imaged at **B**.

(c) Identify and name the portion of the intestinal tract which is imaged at **C**.

(d) Does marker **D** lie on the left or right side of the abdomen? Give reasons for your answer.

(e) Identify and name the region marked **E** and state which bony region it overlies, indicating which bones contribute to this area.

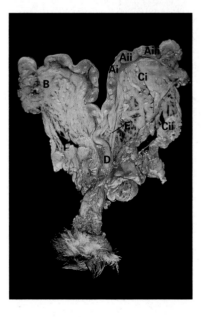

174.

(a) Identify and name the organ and the regions of the organ marked **Ai**, **Aii**, and **Aiii**. Describe the physiological state of this organ giving reasons for your decision.

(b) Identify and name organ **B**, and describe its physiological state. Does your finding help support your answer to question (a)?

(c) Identify and name the tissue folds marked **Ci** and **Cii** and state which structures they attach to in the live dog.

(d) Identify and name the region and the organ marked **D** and state which topographical area it is normally found in.

(e) Identify and name the vessels indicated by marker **E**. If a surgeon wished to remove organ **A**, would it be satisfactory to control haemorrhage by ligating only vessels **E** on each side of the organ? Give reasons for your answer.

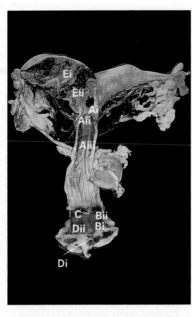

175. This organ has been resected from the abdomen of a bitch and the tubular portion opened to reveal the interior. The contents have been removed.

(a) Identify and name this organ and indicate which portions of the tubular tract are marked **Ai**, **Aii** and **Aiii**.

(b) Identify and name the region of the tract marked **Bi** and indicate the significance of the raised areas of tissue which lie on either side marked **Bii**.

(c) The marker **C** is pointing to an opening in the floor of region **B**. Give a name to this opening and describe what it communicates with and by what means.

(d) Identify and name the structure and region marked **Di** and **Dii**.

(e) Identify and name the region and the organ which has been opened, being marked **Ei** and **Eii**. Comment on the significance of the apparent variation in the colouration of the area.

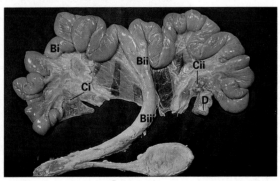

▲ 176.

(a) Identify and name the body system to which these organs belong.

(b) Identify and name the organ and the regions of that organ which are marked **Bi**, **Bii** and **Biii**.

(c) Identify and name the organs which are marked **Ci** and **Cii**. Explain why the surface appearance differs between **Ci** and **Cii**.

(d) Identify and name the tubular structure which is marked **D** and describe what is found at either extremity of it in the live animal.

(e) Using the criteria seen in the previous answers, identify the species and the type of individual shown here giving reasons for your choice.

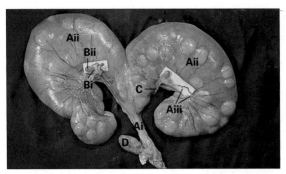

▲ 177.

(a) Identify and name the type of organ and the regions of the organ which are marked **Ai**, **Aii** and **Aiii**. Further identify the rounded structures which can be seen through the outer surface of **Aii**.

(b) Identify and name organ **Bi** and describe the make up and function of structure **Bii** which is apparent on its surface.

(c) Identify and name vessel **C** and state its major vessel of origin. What name is given to the fold of tissue in which it is coursing?

(d) Identify and name organ **D**. What does it contain in life and by which routes does it receive and void its contents?

(e) Using criteria seen in the previous answers, identify the species and the physiological condition of the individual shown, giving your reasons.

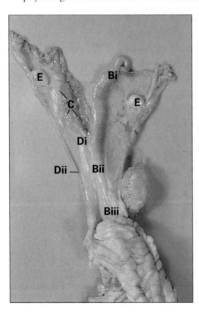

◀ 178.

(a) Identify and name the body system to which this set of organs belongs.

(b) Identify and name the organ and the regions of that organ which are marked **Bi**, **Bii** and **Biii**.

(c) Identify and name the elevated structures which are marked **C** and state what they can be closely related to at certain stages in the animal's life.

(d) Identify and name the fold of tissue which is marked **Di** and specifically name the region of it marked **Dii**.

(e) Identify and name the organ which is marked **E**. Using the criteria seen in this and the previous answers, identify the species involved here, giving your reasons, and comment on the present and past physiological condition of the individual of that species from which the organs were taken.

179. ▶
(a) Identify and name the organ which has been opened here and state which layer of tissues has been exposed by the resection at **A**.
(b) Identify and name the structure which is marked **B** and state what tubular items would be found on opening into it.
(c) Identify and name the structures which are marked **C** and state what they are in close apposition to in the live animal.
(d) Identify and name the structure which is marked **Di** and state what it signifies in relation to the eventual outcome in the development of the creature **Dii**.
(e) The area of tissue marked **E** is overlying a fluid-filled sac. Which sac is this and what is the nature of the material it contains? The fluid-filled sac is directly connected to one of the structures mention in one of the previous answers. Name this structure.

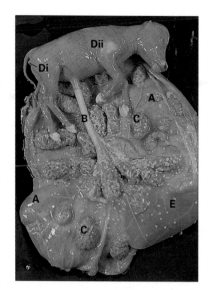

180. ▶ This organ has been removed from the abdominal cavity.
(a) Identify and name the type of organ which is demonstrated here and is marked **A**.
(b) The region of the organ, marked **B**, is being indicated by the insertion of a finger. Name this region.
(c) The region marked **B** has a functional significance to the species involved here. Identify the species and discuss briefly what occurs here at **B**.
(d) The folded tissue which is marked **D** has a specific name and is part of a related structure. Name both of them.
(e) The fold of tissue which is being held at **E** is part of which structure?

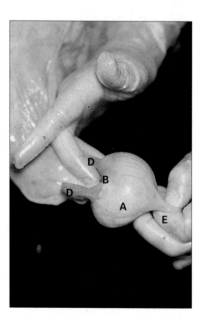

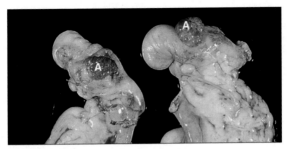

▲ 181. These organs and related structures have been removed from the abdominal cavity.

(a) Identify and name the type of organ which is marked **A**.

(b) Each organ **A** bears on its surface a series of protrusions. Identify what type of structures they represent.

(c) Briefly describe the function of these structures identified in (b).

(d) To reveal the organ **A** a fold of tissue has had to be cut through and pulled back. Identify the fold of tissue and give a name for the enfolding layer it formed as it covered organ **A**.

(e) Using the criteria which you have seen in the previous answers, deduce the species and the physiological state of the individual shown here

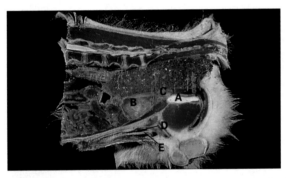

▲ 182. This is a paramedian section of the caudal region of a dog.

(a) Identify and name the structure and region marked **A**.

(b) Identify and name the organ which has been sectioned at **B** and explain how this organ is supported in this position in life.

(c) Identify and name organ **C** and state which other structure it is intimately related to in life. Identify the organ and region of the organ which lies immediately dorsal to **C** and describe the clinical significance of this topographical relationship.

(d) Identify and name the organ and the region of the organ which marker **D** indicates and describe the nature of its composition.

(e) Identify and name structure **E** and describe a related passageway. Give details of this relationship and explain whether possible obstruction of this passageway would occur proximal or distal to **E**.

183. ▶

(a) Identify and name the body system to which these organs belong.

(b) Identify and name the organ marked **B** and state where in the animal's body it would lie in life.

(c) Identify and name the organ marked **C**.

(d) Identify and name the organ marked **D**.

(e) Identify and name the organ marked **E**. Using the criteria seen in this and the previous answers, identify the species and the type of individual shown here, giving your reasons.

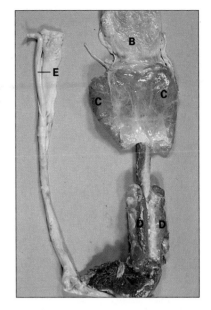

184. ▶

(a) Identify and name the body system to which this organ belongs

(b) Identify and name the organ marked **B**.

(c) Identify and name the region of the organ marked **C**.

(d) Identify and name the opening which is marked **D**.

(e) Using the criteria seen in the previous answers, identify the species shown here, giving your reasons.

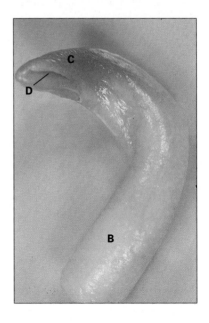

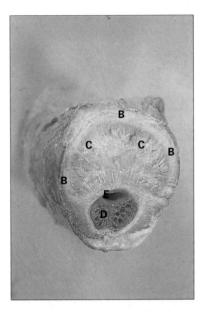

185. This organ has been sectioned transversely to expose the cut face.
(a) Identify and name the type of organ which has been sectioned here.
(b) Identify and name the outer tissue covering which is marked **B**.
(c) Identify and name the region of the organ which is marked **C**
(d) Identify and name the region of the organ which is marked **D**.
(e) Identify and name the cut structure which is seen displayed in cross-section at **E**. What flows through here in life? Using the criteria seen in the previous answers identify the species group into which this organ falls, giving your reasons.

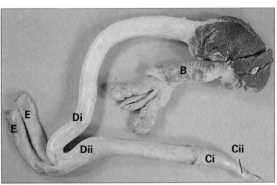

▲ **186.**
(a) Identify and name the body system to which these organs belong.
(b) Identify and name the structure and the region of that structure which is marked **B**.
(c) Identify and name the organ and the region of that organ marked **Ci**. A metal seeker has been inserted into an aperture at **Cii**. Name this aperture and state what it opens into.
(d) Identify and name the region of the organ **C** which lies between the markers **Di** and **Dii**.
(e) Identify and name the structure marked **E**. Using the criteria seen in this and previous answers, identify the species shown here, giving your reasons.

187. ▶

(a) Identify and name organ **Ai**. Name tissue folds **Aii** and identify structures **Aiii** running in them. What did these originally represent?

(b) Identify and name the organs marked **B**. What do they produce and how and where is this product distributed?

(c) If a transverse incision was made through structure **C** at the level of the marker, give the names of the structures which would be encountered on examining the cut face.

(d) Identify and name muscle mass **D**. If a deep transverse incision were made through this muscle at the level of the marker name a glandular structure which might be encountered on examining the cut face.

(e) Identify and name structures **E** and state their function. There is an enlargement of the overall structure at the level of the marker. What name is given to this region? Using the criteria which has been seen so far, name the species, giving your reasons.

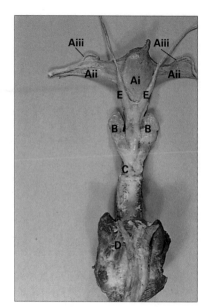

188. ▶ This is the caudolateral aspect of the perineum of a bitch.

(a) Identify and name the bony prominences marked **A** and state which bone they form a part of.

(b) Identify and name muscle **B** and give its origin and insertion.

(c) Identify and name muscle **C** and give its origin and insertion.

(d) Give a collective name and function for structures **B** and **C**.

(e) Identify and name the band of tissue marked **E** and state which structures it connects with.

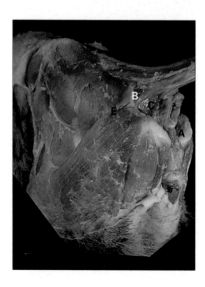

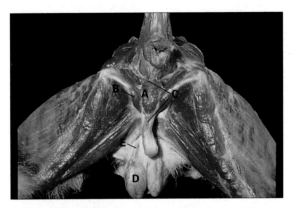

▲ 189. This is the caudal aspect of the perineum of a dog.

(a) Identify and name muscle **A** and state which region of which structure it overlies.

(b) Identify and name muscle **B** and state its origins and insertions.

(c) Identify and name the thin muscle **C**. Which nerve trunk would conduct the motor nerve supply to muscles **A**, **B** and **C**?

(d) Identify and name the organ and its coverings which are marked **D**. State what has been cut away to reveal them.

(e) Identify and name structure **E** and list its contents.

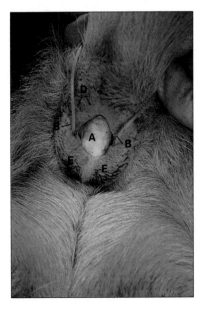

◀ 190.

(a) Identify and name the aperture which bears the cotton plug **A**. State which physical structures control the opening and closing of this aperture in life, giving details of their relative position and composition.

(b) Identify the apertures which are indicated by the tubing marked **B** and describe what they are connected with, giving the precise terminology.

(c) Describe the relationship between the structures in (a) and (b).

(d) The markers **D** are indicating elevations of the surface covering of these regions. What is the significance of the elevations and are they of any clinical significance in the dog? Give details.

(e) What is the source of blood and nerve supply to the surface and deeper structures in the regions marked **E**?

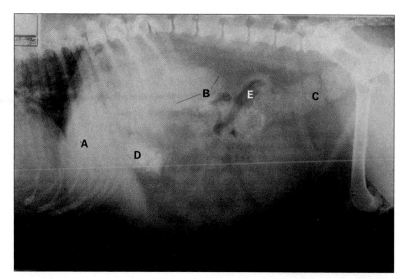

▲ 191.

(a) Identify and name organ **A**.

(b) Identify and name the organ which is indicated as lying between the arrows of marker **B**.

(c) Identify and name the organ and the region of that organ which is indicated as lying in the region marked **C**.

(d) The marker **D** is overlying a dense radio-opaque area which is imaging as whiter than its surroundings. Explain what this image may represent and explain which organ may be involved.

(e) The marker **E** is overlying a radiolucent area which is imaging as darker than its surroundings. Explain this appearance.

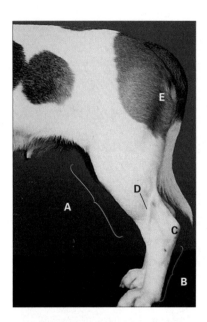

Pelvic Limb

◀ **192.**

(a) State the anatomical regional name for the area marked **A**.

(b) State the anatomical regional name for the area marked **B**.

(c) Identify and name the bony prominence which is palpable at the point marked **C**. Which bone forms this prominence?

(d) Identify and name the structure which is causing this raised elevation of the skin surface at the point marked **D**. Describe the significance of this structure to the clinician.

(e) Identify and name the bony prominence which is palpable in the region marked **E**. Which bone forms this prominence?

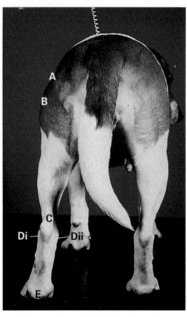

◀ **193.**

(a) Identify and name the bony prominence which can be palpated at **A**. State which bone it forms a part of. Name the muscle mass which attaches in the region of **A**.

(b) Identify and name the muscle mass which lies immediately beneath the skin at region **B**. What is the motor nerve supply to this muscle?

(c) Identify and name the firm band of tissue which could be palpated immediately beneath the skin at region **C**. List the structures which are involved in its composition.

(d) Identify and name the bony prominences which can be palpated at **Di** and **Dii**. Are the two prominences part of the same bone? Explain your answer.

(e) Identify and name the structure which is making ground contact at **E** and state which bony regions it overlies. What is the nerve trunk responsible for conducting cutaneous sensation from this area?

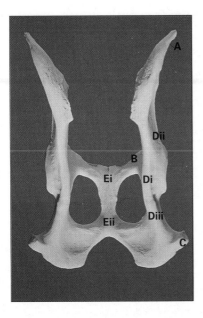

◀194.
(a) Identify and name the bone and the part of this bone marked **A**.
(b) Identify and name the bone and the part of this bone marked **B**.
(c) Identify and name the bone and the part of this bone marked **C**.
(d) Identify and name the bony region marked **Di** and name the depressed areas of bone which lie both cranial, **Dii** and caudal, **Diii**, to it.
(e) Identify and name the bony regions marked **Ei** and **Eii** and state which bones, respectively, contribute to the formation of these areas. Can you form any opinion of the approximate age of this dog from these findings?

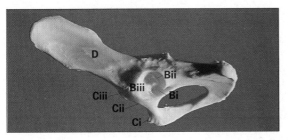

195. ▲
(a) Identify and name this collective bony structure and name the species, with reasons. Which bones make up the total collective specimen?
(b) The marker **Bi** appears to indicate a deficiency in the circular structure marked **Bii** and **Biii**. Give names for the areas and explain the appearance of area **Bi** in the live animal.
(c) Identify and name the regions and the bone marked **Ci**, **Cii** and **Ciii**. Name a tendinous structure which is associated with this area in the live animal and indicate any muscles which can be related to it.
(d) Identify and name the area and the bone marked **D** and indicate the muscles which might attach in this region.
(e) A raised roughened area lies immediately cranial to **Biii**. Which muscle attaches here and what is its action?

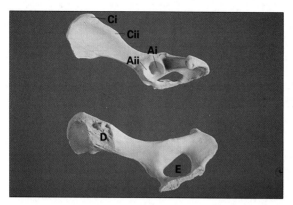

▲ 196.

(a) Identify the regions of bone marked **Ai** and **Aii**. Explain the difference in their surface appearance, giving names.

(b) What structures can be found closely associated with these areas in life?

(c) Identify and name bony eminences **Ci** and **Cii** and state which bone they form a part of. Identify this species, giving reasons for your selection.

(d) Identify and name the region of bone marked **D**. State its functional significance in life. Which bone is this area a part of?

(e) Identify and name aperture **E** and comment on whether it is open in the live dog.

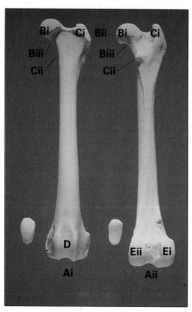

◀ 197.

(a) Identify this bone, giving the species, and state which surfaces of the bone **Ai** and **Aii** indicate.

(b) Identify and name the areas of the bone marked **Bi**, **Bii** and **Biii** and state which structures are closely related to or attached to these areas in the live animal.

(c) Identify and name the areas of bone **Ci** and **Cii** and state which lies medially and which laterally in the live animal. Name both the area of bone lying between them and the raised ridge which connects them distally.

(d) Identify and name area **D** and describe a bony structure which is closely related to it in life. Identify the position of this structure in the slide.

(e) Identify and name areas **Ei** and **Eii**. State what structures these areas are closely related to in life.

198. ▶
(a) Name the muscles which would attach in life to the bony areas marked **Ai**, **Aii** and **Aiii**. What is the action and motor nerve supply of these muscles?
(b) Name the muscles which would attach in life to the bony areas marked **Bi** and **Bii**. What is the action and motor nerve supply of these muscles?
(c) Name the muscles which would attach in life to the bony area marked **C**. What would be the action and motor nerve supply to these muscles?
(d) Name the muscles which would in life attach to the bony areas marked **Di**, **Dii** and **Diii**. What would be the action and motor nerve supply of these muscles?
(e) Name the muscles which would in life attach to the bony area marked **E**. What is the action and motor nerve supply of these muscles?

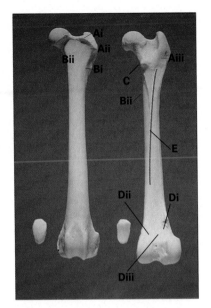

199. ▶
(a) Identify and name the type of bone displayed here.
(b) Identify and name the promontory marked **B**.
(c) Identify and name the region of the bone which is marked **C**.
(d) Identify and name the region of the bone which is marked **D**.
(e) Using the criteria seen in the previous answers, identify the species involved here and whether this bone comes from the left or right limb, giving your reasons.

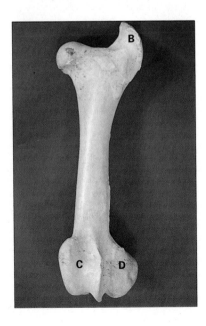

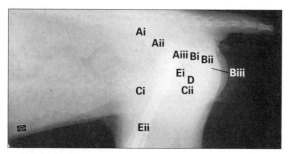

▲ **200.**

(a) Identify and name the bone and the areas of that bone which are marked **Ai, Aii** and **Aiii**.

(b) Identify and name the bone and the areas of that bone which are marked **Bi, Bii** and **Biii**.

(c) Identify and name the bone and the areas of that bone which are marked **Ci** and **Cii**.

(d) Identify and name the area which is imaged as a darkened region marked **D**. Which bones form the edges of this area ?

(e) Identify and name the bone and the areas of that bone marked **Ei** and **Eii**. Can you identify the sex of this animal from the radiograph? Indicate where the evidence lies for your decision.

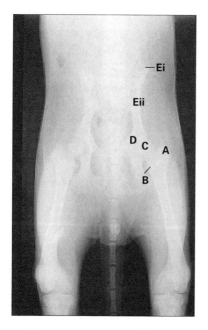

◀ **201.**

(a) Identify and name the bone and region of bone marked **A**.

(b) Identify and name the region of the bone which is marked **B**.

(c) Identify and name the region of bone marked **C** and state which joint it forms a part of. Describe the position the limb is lying in relative to the trunk. How would you describe the movement of the joint that was required to achieve this position?

(d) Identify and name the region which lies immediately to the right of marker **D**. The semicircular outline of this region is not continuous as it appears to have a darker area apparently interrupting the continuity of the semicircle at a position immediately caudal to the marker. Explain this anomaly.

(e) Identify and name the bone and the area of the bone which appears as a whiter line running between the markers **Ei** and **Eii**.

202. ▶

(a) Identify and name the muscle which is marked **A**. Give its origins and insertions, its actions and motor nerve supply.

(b) Identify and name the muscle which is marked **B**. Give its origins and insertions, its action and its motor nerve supply.

(c) Identify and name the muscle which is marked **C**. Give its origins and insertions, its action and its motor nerve supply.

(d) Identify and name the muscles which are marked **Di** and **Dii**. Give their origins and insertions, their actions and their motor nerve supply.

(e) The marker **E** is indicating the union of which two structures? If a longitudinal incision were made here which muscle and which part of which bone would be revealed?

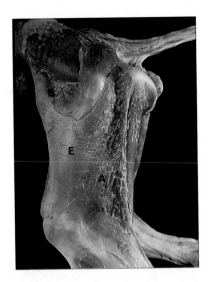

203. ▶

(a) Identify and name the muscle which is marked **Ai** as it lies partially hidden by the larger superficial muscle marked **Aii**. Identify this latter muscle and state whether the two muscles have similar origins, insertions and actions.

(b) Identify and name the muscle marked **B**. Give the origin, insertion and action of this muscle.

(c) Identify and name the muscle marked **C**. Give the origin , insertion and action of this muscle.

(d) Identify and name the muscle marked **D**. Give the origin, insertion and action of this muscle.

(e) If the trunks **Ei** and **Eii** were to be severed separately which of the muscles identified in (a), (b), (c) and (d) would lose their function and which would continue to contract? Identify which area of the limb would be desensitised by such a section.

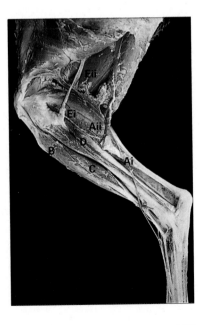

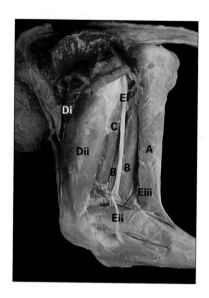

◀ 204.

(a) Identify and name the muscle which is marked **A**. Give its origins and insertions, its action and its motor nerve supply.

(b) Identify and name the muscle which is marked **B**. Give its origins and insertions, its action and its motor nerve supply.

(c) Identify and name the muscle which is marked **C**. Give its origins and insertions, its action and its motor nerve supply.

(d) Identify and name the muscles which are marked **Di** and **Dii**. Give their origins and insertions, their actions and their motor nerve supply.

(e) Identify and name the structure which is marked **Ei**. By following the structure distally, observe its division and name the results of this division marked **Eii** and **Eiii**.

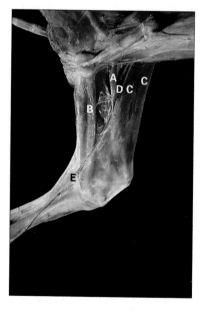

◀ 205.

(a) Identify and name the muscle which is marked **A**. Give the origins and insertions of this muscle along with its action and motor nerve supply.

(b) Identify and name the muscle which is marked **B**. Give the origins and insertions of the muscle along with its actions and motor nerve supply.

(c) Identify and name the muscle which is marked **C**. Give the origins and insertions of the muscle along with its actions and motor nerve supply.

(d) Identify and name the region which is marked **D** and state which major vascular and neurological structures run through this region. Of what significance is this region to the examining clinician?

(e) Identify and name the vessel marked **E** and state in which direction blood is flowing in it.

206. ▶

(a) Identify and name the muscle which is marked **A**. Give the origins and insertions of the muscle along with its action and motor nerve supply.

(b) Identify and name the muscle which is marked **B**. Give the origins and insertions of the muscle along with its action and motor nerve supply.

(c) Identify and name the muscle which is marked **C**. Give its origins and insertions commenting on all its bony connections. What are its actions and motor nerve supply?

(d) Identify and name the landmarks which are indicated at **Di**, **Dii** and **Diii** explaining the interconnections formed between them.

(e) The marker **E** is overlying a longitudinally running structure which appears to have multiple components. Elaborate on these comments giving names.

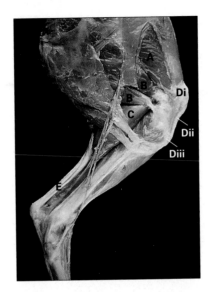

207. ▶

(a) Identify and name the bones which are displayed in this photograph and describe which aspects of these bones are being viewed in **Ai** and **Aii**.

(b) Identify and name the areas of the bone marked **Bi** and **Bii**. In life which structures would be closely applied to these surfaces?

(c) Identify and name the areas of the bone marked **Ci**, **Cii**, **Ciii** and **Civ**. Name any ligamentous structures which may be related to these areas in the live animal.

(d) Identify and name the area of the bone marked **D** and state what major attachment may be made here in life.

(e) Identify and name the areas of these bones which are marked **Ei** and **Eii** and state what ligamentous structures may attach here in life.

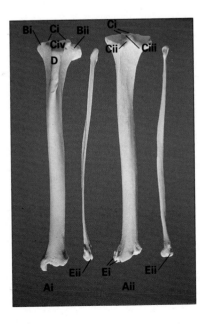

107

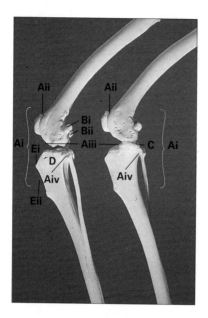

◀ **208.**

(a) Identify the joint which is marked **Ai** and name the subdivisions of the joint which are marked **Aii**, **Aiii** and **Aiv** describing the articular surfaces of each.

(b) Identify and name the structures which are marked **Bi** and **Bii** and state with which soft tissue structures they are closely related in life and what purpose they serve.

(c) Identify and name the structure marked **C** and state with which soft tissue structure it is closely related in life.

(d) Identify and name the groove which is apparent on the bony surface at **D** and state which structure passes through this groove in life. Is this groove lying on the lateral or medial aspect of the bone?

(e) Identify and name the bony eminences which are marked **Ei** and **Eii**. How is **Ei** formed in the young animal and name any muscles which insert at **Ei** and **Eii**.

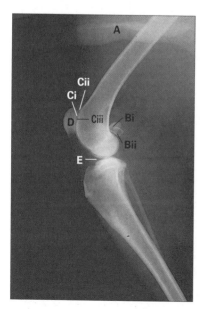

◀ **209.**

(a) Identify and name the structure which is marked **A**.

(b) Identify and name the structures which are imaged at **Bi** and **Bii** and relate their functional significance in life.

(c) Identify the linear images on the bone surface which are marked **Ci**, **Cii** and **Ciii**.

(d) Identify and name the bone marked **D** and state how it relates to the structures **Ci**, **Cii** and **Ciii** during movement of this joint.

(e) The marker **E** is indicating an apparent space. Is this a true space in the live animal? Which movements can be expected here under normal conditions?

210. ▶
(a) Identify and name the type of bones displayed here.
(b) Identify and name the area marked **Bi** and give the terms used for the peaks of bone marked **Bii** and **Biii**.
(c) Identify and name the areas of bone marked **Ci** and **Cii**.
(d) Identify and name the area of bone marked **D**.
(e) Using the criteria seen in the previous answers, identify the species involved here and state whether the bone is from a left or right limb, giving your reasons.

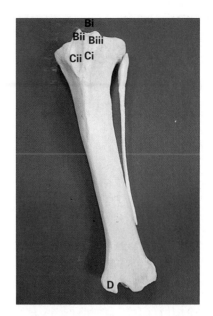

211. ▶
(a) Identify and name the bone which is marked **A**.
(b) Identify the bone and the region of that bone which is outlined by the markers **B**. Using the criteria seen in this and the previous answer, identify the species involved here, giving your reasons.
(c) Identify and name the regions of the bone which are marked **C** and state what they come into contact with in life.
(d) Identify and name the prominence marked **D** and state what attaches here in life.
(e) Identify the darkened area marked **E** and give reasons for its lack of density.

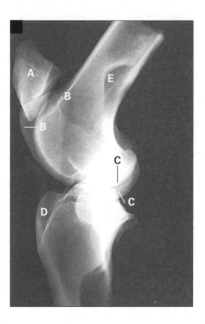

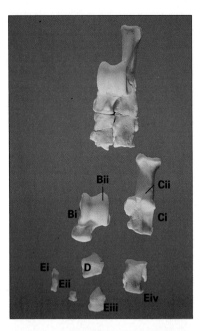

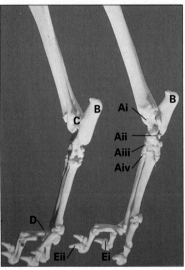

◀ 212.
(a) Identify the collective gathering of
bones exhibited in the top region of
the photograph and indicate which
aspect of these bones is being viewed
here.
(b) Identify the bone marked **Bi** and the
area of that bone marked **Bii**.
(c) Identify and name the bone marked
Ci and the shelf-like area of bone
marked **Cii**.
(d) Identify and name the bone marked
D. With which other bones of the
series does it articulate and on which
of its faces are these articulations?
(e) The bones **Ei**, **Eii**, **Eiii** and **Eiv** are
arranged serially. Which is most medial
and which most lateral in the live
animal?

◀ 213.
(a) Identify and name the specific joints
marked **Ai**, **Aii**, **Aiii** and **Aiv**. Which of
these joints experiences the greatest
degree of movement during movement
of the total area and what type of
movements are seen here in life?
(b) Identify and name the bone and the
region of that bone which is marked
B. What attaches here in life and how
is this region formed in the young
animal?
(c) Identify and name the promontory
marked **C** and state which bone it
belongs to. Name which ligamentous
structure attaches here and describe its
format and other attachments.
(d) Identify and name the small bony
structure which is marked **D** and
describe how it maintains this position
in the live animal.
(e) Identify and name the bone and the
portions of that bone marked **Ei** and
Eii. What covers these regions in life?

110

214. ▶

(a) Identify by number and name the bones marked **A**. What type of bones are these and how do they develop in the immature animal?

(b) In life which muscular structures are found closely applied to the plantar surfaces of the bones marked **A**? How and where do these muscles insert?

(c) Identify and name the structures marked **C** and relate what structures hold them in this position in the live animal.

(d) In the live animal, which tendinous structures are found running over the space existing between the structures marked **C**? What holds them in this space?

(e) Identify and name the sequence of bones marked **E**. What type of bones are they and how do they develop in the immature animal?

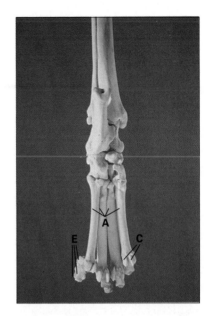

215. ▶

(a) Identify and name the joint space which is imaged at **A**.

(b) Identify and name the bone which is imaged at **B**.

(c) Identify the bone which is imaged at **Ci** and name the portion of it which is marked **Cii**.

(d) Identify and name the bone which is marked **D** and state whether it is lying on the medial or lateral side of the limb.

(e) Identify and name the joint space which is marked at **Ei** and comment on the significance of the oval white images which appear immediately proximal to this joint, **Eii**, and to the same joints in the other digits.

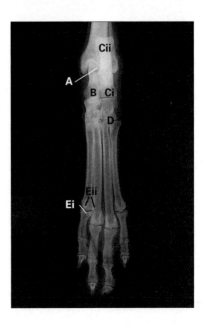

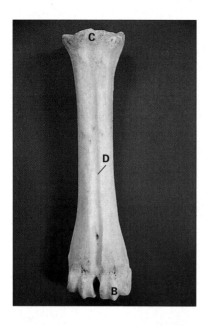

◄216.

(a) Identify and name the type of bone displayed here.

(b) Identify and name the region of the bone marked **B** and state with which region of which bone it is closely associated in the live animal.

(c) Identify the raised area of bone marked **C** and state what attaches here in the live animal.

(d) Comment on the significance of the groove which is apparent on the bone surface and is marked **D**. Which aspect of the bone is shown here?

(e) Using the criteria seen in the previous answers, state your reasons for identifying the species involved here.

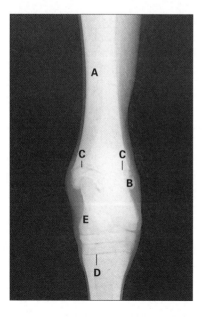

◄217.

(a) Identify and name the bone which is marked **A**.

(b) Identify and name the structure which is marked **B**. State what it represents and whether it is a normal feature of this region. Identify the species involved.

(c) The markers **C** are pointing to a dark line. What does it represent?

(d) The marker **D** is pointing to a dark line. What does it represent?

(e) Identify and name the bone marked **E**. Does the marker lie to the medial or lateral side of the region?

218. ▶

(a) Identify and name the bone and the region of that bone marked **A**.

(b) Identify and name the bone marked **Bi** and state what the edge marked **Bii** represents.

(c) Identify and name the bone marked **C**.

(d) Identify and name the bone marked **D**.

(e) Identify and name the bones marked **Ei** and **Eii** and state which lies medially in the live animal. Which species is this? Give reasons for your decisions.

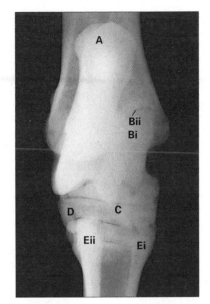

219. ▶

(a) Identify and name the structure which is marked **A**. In general terms, where does it originate from and on what structures does it insert? Give the species involved here.

(b) Identify and name the structure marked **B**. Which region does it originate from and how does it terminate?

(c) Identify and name the structure which is marked **C**. Which area does it originate from and where does it terminate?

(d) Identify and name the structure which is marked **D**. In general terms, where does it originate from and how does it terminate?

(e) Identify and name the structure which is marked **Ei**. In general terms, where does it originate from and what does it terminate on? What is happening to this structure at the level marked **Eii**?

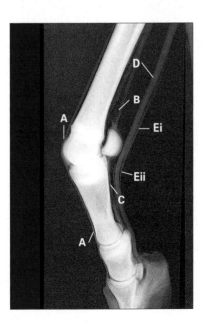

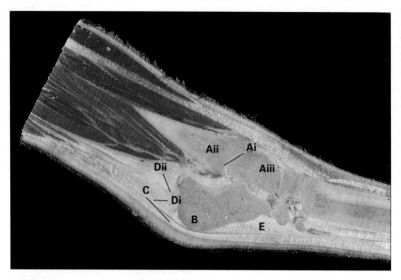

▲ 220.

(a) Identify the joint space which is marked **Ai** and name the bones which make the articulation, marked **Aii** and **Aiii**.

(b) Identify and name the bone and the region of that bone which is marked **B**.

(c) Identify and name structure **C** which has been sectioned in the long axis. State where it originates and terminates.

(d) Identify and name the structure **Di** which has been sectioned in long axis. Describe the nature of the structure which occupies the area which is marked **Dii**.

(e) Identify and name the structure which has been sectioned at **E**. What is its function in the live animal? Describe its attachments.

Gross Anatomy

1. (a) Arrow **Ai** is pointing in a cranial direction while arrow **Aii** is directed in a caudal direction.
   (b) The terms would be different for **Bi** because this should be rostral as it is being applied in the region which is already cranial. **Bii** is still termed caudal.
   (c) **Ci** and **Cii** could be called cranial and caudal, respectively, but **Ciii** and **Civ** are termed dorsal and palmar as they refer to the distal thoracic limb. **Cv** and **Cvi** are termed dorsal and plantar, respectively, because they refer to the distal pelvic limb. The terms cranial and caudal do not apply distally because that portion of the limb is so mobile it would be difficult to constantly relate it to the cranium or tail of the animal.
   (d) **Di** refers to the dorsal region while **Dii** indicates the ventral region.
   (e) **Ei** is the lateral aspect of the limb as opposed to **Eii** which indicates the medial aspect.

2. (a) **Ai**— cervical vertebrae (7), **Aii** — thoracic vertebrae (13), **Aiii** — lumbar vertebrae (7) and **Aiv** — sacral vertebrae (3 in number but fused into a single unit).
   (b) **Bi** — scapula, **Bii** — humerus, **Biii** — radius and ulna, **Biv** — carpus.
   (c) **Ci** — ossa coxae, **Cii** — femur, **Ciii** — tibia and fibula, **Civ** — tarsus.
   (d) This is the sternum which is composed of eight elements. The most cranial is the manubrium and the most caudal is the xiphoid.
   (e) **Ei** indicates the metacarpal bones, potentially five in each manus but the first digit may have been removed shortly after birth leaving only four. **Eii** is indicating the metatarsal bones. Most dogs have only four present in each pes but there may be a vestigial first digit in some breeds and individuals with a rudimentary first metatarsal bone. In the Pyreenean Mountain Dog there is commonly a duplicate rudimentary first digit in each pes.

Head and Neck

3. (a) This is the median plane as it traverses exactly through the midline axis of the body. Aii indicates a section in the sagittal plane as it traverses from cranial to caudal, parallel to the midline axis of the body.
   (b) This is the axial plane as the line traverses through the axis of the thoracic limb.
   (c) The direction indicated by **Ci** is abaxial as opposed to **Cii** which is axial.
   (d) The direction indicated by **Di** is proximal as opposed to the direction of **Dii** which is distal.
   (e) This is the cranial aspect of the dog but if it turned around we would see the caudal aspect.

4. (a) The larynx lies subcutaneously at point A. The most ventral point of the larynx is the body of the thyroid cartilage.
   (b) Point **B** would overlie the external occipital protuberance of the occipital bone
   (c) Point **C** identifies the puncta lacrimale of the lower lid, which is situated at the medial commissure of the eyelids. The lacrimal secretions drain through this orifice.
   (d) This site overlies the m. masseter over which, at point **D**, would run the dorsal buccal branches of the facial (VII) nerve. Section of these nerves would result in loss of motor function to some muscles of facial expression on the lateral side of the face. The duct of the parotid salivary gland also runs in this position carrying salivary secretion to the oral cavity. Laceration could interfere with this flow.
   (e) Point **E** is the site for venipunture involving the external jugular vein.

ANSWERS

5. (a) Structure **A** is the third eyelid lying at the medial commissure of the eyelids. It has a protective function being capable of passing over the bulbar conjunctiva as the ocular bulb is drawn caudally by retraction of the eyeball into the orbit.

(b) The palpable area is the zygomatic arch which is formed by the temporal bone caudally, the zygomatic bone itself and the maxilla cranially.

(c) The aperture which may be palpated is the infraorbital canal opening, the infraorbital foramen could be palpated here in the maxilla.

(d) The zygomatic process of the frontal bone is found at point **D**. This gives attachment to the orbital ligament which runs to the temporal process of the zygomatic bone providing a lateral boundary to the orbital rim.

(e) Aperture **E** identifies an external naris beyond which one enters into the vestibule, the nasal meatuses extend from the vestibule.

6. (a) Point **A** marks the temporomandibular joint which is a condylar joint.

(b) The articular surfaces are normally formed by the condylar process of the mandible and the mandibular fossa of the temporal bone. There is an articular disc of fibrocartilage lying between the two adjacent surfaces.

(c) Bony prominence **C** is the angular process of the mandible which gives attachment to the mms. pterygoideus medially and the m. masseter laterally.

(d) The action of the muscles in (c) is flexion of the temporomandibular joint and therefore closure of the mouth. Motor innervation is by the trigeminal (V) nerve.

(e) Tooth **E** is the carnassial tooth or fourth premolar of the upper jaw. It functions as the sectorial tooth of the upper dental arcade and has a trifid root system which usually necessitates surgical removal by elevation from its alveolus rather than by straight traction.

7. (a) This area is the parietal bone of the skull of a cat which overlies the cranial cavity.

(b) The marker indicates the zygomatic process of the frontal bone.

(c) Prominence **C** is the frontal process of the zygomatic bone. **B** and **C** are joined in life by the orbital ligament.

(d) The marker indicates the fossa for the lacrimal sac in the lacrimal bone. The lacrimal caniculi run into the sac at this point.

(e) The markers indicate the mental foramina of the body of the mandible through which run the mental nerves. These nerves are branches of the trigeminal (V) nerve coming from the inferior alveolar nerve within the mandibular canal.

8. (a) This is the skull of a cat, sectioned in the sagittal plane extremely close to the median axis. The photograph is displaying the medial aspect of this section of skull.

(b) Structure **B** is the tentorium osseum which separates the cerebellum from the cerebral hemispheres.

(c) Depression **C** is the dorsum sellae which houses the hypophysis cerebri in life.

(d) Aperture **D** is the opening of the optic canal which allows passage to the optic (II) nerve.

(e) The bony areas are as follows: **Ei** — dorsal nasal conchae and **Eii** — ventral nasal conchae. The middle meatus communicates with the common meatus of the nasal passageway between these areas.

9. (a) Bone **A** is the frontal bone in the skull of an adult cat.
   (b) Bone **B** is the occipital bone. This would surround the opening of the foramen magnum.
   (c) Bone **C** is the parietal bone which would overlie the cerebral hemispheres.
   (d) Bone **D** is the incisive bone which bears the incisor teeth, three in each bone.
   (e) Bone **E** is the maxilla. This bone also has a ventral and medial portion which forms part of the hard palate.

10. (a) Area **A** is the frontal sinus, an air-filled recess within the frontal bone. There is only a thin plate of bone overlying this air space and it images as a darker area of reduced radio-opacity.
   (b) Structure **B** is the hard palate, separating the ventrally placed oral cavity from the ventral meatus of the nasal cavity dorsally.
   (c) Area **C** is the external acoustic meatus leading from the exterior of the skull to the middle ear. The meatus is air filled and is imaged superimposed over the air filled tympanic bulla which surrounds it ventrally. This produces an area of reduced radio-opacity.
   (d) The fine line imaged at **D** is the epihyoid bone. It is part of the hyoid apparatus which forms a bony base for the root (radix) of the tongue.
   (e) Point **E** is the root of the upper canine tooth. This tooth is implanted in the maxilla.

11. (a) Apertures **A** are the palatine fissures. Each fissure lies at the junction between the incisive bone and maxilla and gives passage to an incisive duct (nasopalatine duct) which passes from the oral cavity to the nasal cavity communicating with the vomeronasal organ.
   (b) Structures **B** are two molar teeth of the upper dental arcade. These teeth are implanted in the maxilla and are used for crushing food. The first and second molars each have three roots.
   (c) Aperture **C** is the hypoglossal canal which gives passage to the hypoglossal nerve. It is located in the occipital bone of the skull.
   (d) Aperture **D** is the foramen magnum which permits passage of the spinal cord from the cranium to the vertebral canal along with the surrounding meningeal layers and blood vessels.
   (e) Aperture **E** is the foramen ovale which allows passage of the mandibular branch of the trigeminal (V) nerve.

12. (a) Bone **A** is the basisphenoid bone which articulates rostrally with the presphenoid bone and caudally with the basioccipital bone.
   (b) Structures **B** indicate the tympanic bullae of the temporal bones of the skull.
   (c) Aperture **C** is the mandibular fossae of the temporal bones. These are for articulation of the condyloid processes of the mandible with a fibrocartilage disc interposed between them.
   (d) Markers **D** indicate the zygomatic bone which forms part of the zygomatic arch.
   (e) Aperture **E** is the opening of the alveolus of the canine tooth. The space is occupied by the root of the canine tooth which is attached by the periodontal ligament, running from the cementum of the tooth to the alveolar bone. This forms a type of joint — a gomphosis.

ANSWERS

13.(a) Bony eminence **A** is the occipital condyle (condyloid process) of the occipital bone of a cat. The condyle makes an articulation with the cranial articular fovea of the atlas (first cervical vertebra).

(b) Structure **B** is the hamulus of the pterygoid bone which gives the origin to the m. pterygoideus medialis and the m. pterygopharyngeus tendon. The m. tensor veli palatini passes over this area on a trochlear ridge.

(c) Aperture **C** is the opening of the alar canal, i.e. the caudal alar foramen which lies in the sphenoid bone. The maxillary branch of the trigeminal (V) nerve would pass through it in life.

(d) Structure **D** is a molar tooth of the upper dental arcade. The tooth immediately rostral to it is the fourth premolar which is the carnassial or sectorial tooth of the cat. The presence of **D** indicates an adult cat as the molar tooth is not represented in the temporary dentition.

(e) The coloured line is the palatomaxillary suture. This was the growth area between the palatine bone and the maxilla in the immature skull, this is now calcified indicating the skull of a mature cat.

14.(a) These bones constitute the left and right and articulated mandibles.

(b) Area **B** is the medial aspect of the ramus of the left mandible.

(c) The non-bony structures are, from rostral to caudal, three incisor teeth, a single canine tooth, two premolar teeth and a single molar tooth.

(d) The dentition is characteristic of an adult cat. An adult dog would have four premolar and three molar teeth in the lower dental arcade.

(e) Aperture **E** is the mandibular foramen. Entering through it is the mandibular alveolar artery which is given off from the maxillary artery just before the point of entry.

15.(a) Bone **A** is the frontal bone and the projection lying on the lateral edge of each side is the zygomatic process (supraorbital process).

(b) Bone projection **B** is the angular process of the body of the mandible. Attaching here are the m. masseter laterally and the m. pterygoideus medialis medially. These muscles cause closure of the mouth on contraction, they are innervated by the mandibular branch of the trigeminal (V) nerve.

(c) Region **C** is the mandibular symphysis. This area represents the joint formed between the two mandibular bodies and consists of fibrocartilaginous material representing a synchondrosis. The fibrocartilage persists throughout life and so the structure is a constant feature in both young and old dogs.

(d) Aperture **D** is the infraorbital foramen in the maxilla. The infraorbital nerve, derived from the maxillary branch of the trigeminal (V) nerve, passes through it. This nerve is responsible for innervation of the premolar and incisor teeth and the nasal region. The infraorbitol nerve is accompanied by the infraorbital artery and vein which supply the rostral nasal region. The artery is a continuation of the maxillary artery while the vein connects with the facial vein and the deeper venous drainage in the pterygopalatine fossa. These vessels provide vascular supply and drainage of the rostral nasal region.

(e) Apertures **E** are the mental foramina in the mandibular bodies, which give passage to the mental nerves from the inferior alveolar nerve which, in turn, arises from the mandibular branch of the trigeminal (V) nerve. The nerves supply the rostral premolar and incisor teeth and the lower mental region.

16. (a) Surface **A** is the cranial articular surface of the second cervical vertebra (axis).
    (b) Area **B** is the transverse process of the first cervical vertebra (atlas).
    (c) Prominence **C** is the mastoid process of the temporal bone.
    (d) Area **D** marks the ethmoturbinates of the ethmoid bone.
    (e) These structures are canine teeth, **Ei** is an upper canine, **Eii** is a lower canine. The lower canine lies rostral to the upper in the serial row of occluded teeth.

17. (a) Teeth **A** are the incisor teeth of the upper and lower dental arcades. The first pair of teeth, central incisors, are placed most medially in the rostral region of the incisive bone while the third pair of teeth, lateral incisors, are situated most laterally in the same bone.
    (b) Teeth **B** are the first premolar teeth of the upper and lower jaw. These teeth are difficult to define in terms of eruption as they arise at the time of the temporary dentition but remain with the permanent dentition without being shed or replaced.
    (c) Teeth **C** are the canine teeth of the upper and lower arcades. These are the teeth of offence being designed to puncture and kill. The lower canine tooth lies more rostrally when viewed in the live dog with its upper and lower arcades closed in apposition.
    (d) Tooth marker **Di** shows a root covered in cementum; **Dii** shows an apex, through which passes the nutrient blood vessels and the nerve trunks; **Diii** indicates the neck, where the mucous membrane of the gum meets the tooth surface; **Div** shows the crown, covered in enamel.
    (e) Tooth **E** is the fourth upper premolar tooth, which is also called the sectorial or carnassial tooth due to its function of shearing the food as it is moved laterally into a position between the fourth upper premolar and the first lower molar. Abcessation of the root would cause swelling of the facial region or even fistulation (discharge) rostroventral to the eye.

18. (a) Teeth **A** are incisor teeth.
    (b) Teeth **B** are canine teeth.
    (c) Teeth **C** are premolar teeth.
    (d) Teeth **D** are molar teeth.
    (e) This is the complete dental arcade from an adult cat. Molar teeth are present which makes it an adult dentition. The sharp pointed canines are indicative of a cat and the formula of Pm3/2; M1/1 is characteristic of the cat compared with Pm4/4; M2/3 of a dog.

19. (a) Structures **A** are the incisor teeth. There appears to be four on each half of the dental arcade which is an unusual feature. It is postulated that the lateral incisor is, in fact, the migrated and modified canine tooth.
    (b) Areas **B** are the lateral walls of the buccal vestibules or cheeks. These are covered with cone-shaped cornified papillae.
    (c) Markers **C** are the sublingual caruncles onto which open the mandibular salivary duct and the major sublingual salivary duct from the monostomatic portion of the sublingual salivary gland.
    (d) The apparent presence of four incisor teeth and conical papillae of the cheek indicates a ruminant.
    (e) The tongue has been removed by the section of the m. genioglossus muscle at each side marked **Eii**.

20. (a) Marker **A** indicates the m. orbicularis oris which moves and closes the lips.

(b) Muscle **B** is the m. masseter which originates in the maxillary region of the skull and the zygomatic arch and inserts onto the masseteric fossa of the mandible.

(c) Muscle **C** is the m. digastricus which originates from the paracondylar process of the occiput and inserts on the ventral mandibular border.

(d) Marker **D** shows the dorsal buccal branch of the facial (VII) nerve. Its section would produce loss of function of the m. orbicularis oris and the caudal portion of the m. diagastricus as the motor nerve supply is by the mandibular branch of the trigeminal (V) nerve to the rostral portion and facial (VII) nerve to the caudal portion.

(e) Structure **E** is the parotid salivary gland. The parotid duct passes rostrally, running over the lateral aspect of the masseter muscle, to open into the oral cavity and dorsally in the buccal cavity (opposite the fourth upper premolar tooth).

21. (a) Muscle **A** is the m. buccinator, which is responsible for tensing the buccal or cheek region and moving food back onto the masticatory surface of the molar teeth. This muscle's motor nerve supply is from the buccal branches of the facial (VII) nerve.

(b) Muscle **B** is the m. digastricus which plays a part in opening the mouth. When acting bilaterally and lateral deviation of the lower jaw with unilateral contraction. It has a dual nerve supply by the trigeminal (V) and facial (VII) nerves.

(c) Muscle **C** is the m. temporalis which plays a part in closure of the jaw. It has a motor nerve supply from the trigeminal (V) nerve.

(d) Marker **D** lies over the m. thyropharyngeus which belongs to the pharyngeal group of muscles which produce constriction of the pharynx. The motor nerve supply is through the glossopharyngeal (IX) and vagus (X) nerves.

(e) The markers lie over the heads of origin of the m. sternocephalicus muscle which are from the mastoid area of the temporal bone and the occipital region of the skull. This muscle produces lateral side-to-side movements of the head and neck and is innervated by ventral branches of cervical spinal nerves and the accessory (XI) nerve.

22. (a) Structures **A** are the mandibular lymph nodes. There are several structures involved in this group of nodes and they lie on both sides of the facial vein.

(b) Structure **B** is the mandibular salivary gland. This appears as a single structure but in fact incorporates two portions of salivary gland tissue, the mandibular gland proper and the monostomatic portion of the sublingual salivary gland, both within the same capsule. The encapsulated structure lies on the V formed by the facial vein and the maxillary vein.

(c) Vessel **C** is the external jugular vein. This originates from the union of the linguofacial vein and the maxillary vein and terminates by joining the subclavian vein and running into the cranial vena cava.

(d) Muscle **D** is the m. sternohyoideus which runs from the basihyoid bone to the manubrium of the sternum. This muscle retracts the hyoid apparatus during swallowing.

(e) Muscle **Ei** is the m. cleidomastoideus and **Eii** is the m. cleidocervicalis. These fuse at the clavicular tendon to continue as the m. cleidobrachialis (**Eiii**). These muscles are collectively known as the m. brachiocephalicus. Acting unilaterally, they cause lateral deviation of the head and neck when the thoracic limb is fixed or protraction of the thoracic limb and extension of shoulder joint during locomotion. Acting bilaterally with the limbs fixed, they produce a ventral flexion of the neck. Their motor nerve supply is by the spinal accessory nerve (XI) to **Ei** and **Eii**. Muscle **Eiii** is supplied by the axillary nerve.

23. (a) The sectioned muscle is the m. masseter which plays a part in closure of the mouth.

(b) Muscle **B** is the m. sternohyoideus which assists in pulling the basihyoid and the tongue caudally.

(c) Muscle **C** is the m. styloglossus which, acting bilaterally, assists in retracting the tongue and unilaterally in lateral deviation of the tongue.

(d) Muscle **D** is the m. hyoglossus which, acting bilaterally, assists in retracting the tongue and unilaterally in lateral deviation of the tongue.

(e) Structure **E** is the hypoglossal nerve. If it were sectioned it would affect the muscle contraction of **C** and **D** but the m. masseter receives a motor nerve supply from the trigeminal (V) nerve and the m. sternohyoideus receives supply from the cervical nerves and the accessory nerve so these would be unaffected.

24. (a) Space **A** is the maxillary recess of the maxilla.

(b) Space **B** is the infraorbital canal cut in cross section. This contains the infraorbital nerve (which is derived from the maxillary branch of the trigeminal (V) nerve) and the infraorbital artery and vein.

(c) Space **C** is the choana leading to the nasopharyngeal meatus which connects with the nasopharynx; its ventral margin is formed by the palatine bone.

(d) Marker **D** indicates the vomer bone which forms the ventral support to the nasal septum.

(e) Bone **E** is the ethmoid bone. The perpendicular plate or lamina is seen ventral to the marker while the lateral lamina is situated more lateral to it.

25. (a) Area **A** is the osseous nasal septum of the ethmoid bone. This is continued rostrally by the membranous and cartilaginous portions of the nasal septum as far as the external nares.

(b) Bone area **B** is the median septum of the frontal sinus, part of the frontal bone. Sectioned on the median plane as if it were paramedian, the air space of the frontal sinus would be revealed.

(c) Area **C** is the body of the basisphenoid bone. The area dorsal to it is the region of the hypophyseal fossa which, in life, accommodates the hypophysis cerebri.

(d) Area **D** is the tentorium osseum which principally comprises the leaves of bone from the parietal bones, although the internal occipital protuberance of the occipital bone also contributes to its formation. The shelf of bone thus formed projects between the cerebral hemispheres and the cerebellum at the line of the transverse fissure.

(e) Bone **E** is the vomer bone which forms the caudoventral part of the nasal septum. The vomer bone is associated with the sphenoid, ethmoid, palatine and incisive bones, in addition to the maxilla.

26. (a) Marker **A** shows the parietal bone, a flat bone overlying the cerebral hemispheres of the brain as they occupy the dorsal portion of the cranial cavity of the skull.

(b) Markers **Bi** and **Bii** show the dorsal and ventral nasal conchae, between which normally lies the middle meatus.

(c) Marker **C** shows the cribriform plate of the ethmoid bone. The caudal face is associated with the olfactory bulbs of the brain, multiple foramina allowing passage of fibres from the olfactory nerve.

(d) Respectively, the markers indicate the petrosal and tympanic parts of the temporal bone. Thus, these areas are portions of the same bone.

ANSWERS

(e) Marker **E** shows the nasopharyngeal meatus through which air moves during respiration. Food is prevented from being projected through this passageway into the nasal cavity from the pharyngeal cavity by the presence of the soft palate. The latter is suspended ventral and caudal to the caudal opening of the passageway.

27. (a) The regions are as follows: **Ai** — cerebral hemisphere, **Aii** — cerebellum.
(b) The regions are as follows: **Bi** — the pons, **Bii** — the medulla oblongata.
(c) The markers are as follows: **Ci** — nasopharynx, **Cii** — soft palate, **Ciii** — epiglottis.
(d) This tissue is the vocal fold which attaches to the vocal process of the arytenoid cartilage dorsally and the thyroid cartilage ventrally.
(e) This is the opening of the lateral ventricle which is found lying between the vocal fold caudally and the vestibular fold rostrally.

28. (a) The marker indicates the frontal sinus, which is found in frontal bone.
(b) This space is the palatine sinus of the palatine bone and maxilla.
(c) This space is the aditus laryngis. The epiglottis lies cranioventrally while the corniculate processes of arytenoids lie dorsally, the aryepiglottic folds run on either side.
(d) The markers are as follows: **Di** — ventral meatus, **Dii** — ventral nasal concha.
(e) The markers are as follows: **Ei** — joint space of atlanto-axial joint, **Eii** — atlas, **Eiii** — axis.

29. (a) This group is the m. temporalis which acts to produce closure of the mouth and is innervated by the maxillary branch of the trigeminal (V) nerve.
(b) Structure **B** is the cerebral hemisphere of the brain, the cut surface of which exhibits a variation of grey and white matter. The grey matter is more peripheral and represents the non-myelinated grey matter consisting of cell bodies and nuclei while the more centrally placed white matter is the myelinated area of the nerve fibre tracts.
(c) Structure **C** is the lens of the eye which is maintained in position by fixation through the zonular fibres, zonula ciliaris and the ciliary body which lies peripheral to it in this section.
(d) Region **D** is the vitreous chamber of the eye which contains the vitreous body in life.
(e) The openings marked are (caudally) the lacrimal sac, the starting point of the nasolacrimal duct, and (rostrally) the opening of that duct onto the ventrolateral floor of the nasal vestibule below the alar fold.

30. (a) Marker **A** shows the cornea of the eyeball, the rostral surface of which is covered by bulbar conjunctiva.
(b) Marker **B** shows the posterior chamber of the eyeball which, in life, is filled with aqueous fluid which flows through the opening of the pupil from the anterior chamber.
(c) Layer **C** is the sclera which meets the cornea at the region called the limbus corneae.
(d) Surface **D** is the periorbita, a fibrous layer which forms a lining for the bony orbit of the skull.
(e) The marker **Ei** is pointing to the m. retractor bulbi (which pulls the eyeball deeper into the orbit) while **Eii** is indicating the m. recti medialis and the m. obliquus dorsalis (which produce rotational movements of the eyeball). The retractor is supplied by the abducent (VI) nerve, the lateral rectus by the oculomotor (III) nerve and dorsal oblique by the trochlear (IV) nerve.

31. (a) Structure **A** is the epiglottis which predominantly consists of elastic cartilage. The epiglottis is the most rostral cartilage of the larynx.

(b) Structure **B** is the palatine tonsil which is lying partially hidden in its crypt. It is part of the defence mechanism of the body, containing lymphatic tissue.

(c) Structure **C** is the oral surface of the soft palate. This curtain-like flap of tissue extends caudally into the pharynx dividing the oropharynx from the nasopharynx.

(d) Marker **D** indicates the dorsal surface of the body of the tongue. The rounded structures are vallate papillae, which function as taste buds.

(e) The tissue fold is the palatoglossal arch, which bears filiform papillae on its surface. These papillae have a mechanical function assisting in holding food on the tongue's surface.

32. (a) Region **A** is the dental pad. The appearance of a rostral region is indicative of a ruminant species as these animals lack upper incisor teeth.

(b) Region **Bi** is the hard palate, which is based upon the maxillae and the palatine bones. **Bii** indicates the palatine raphe.

(c) Region **C** is the soft palate which comes into contact with the epiglottis along its caudal edge.

(d) Structure **D** is an incisive papilla which has openings of the incisive ducts.

(e) Space **E** is the buccal vestibule which has molar and premolar teeth lying medially and muscles of the cheek lying laterally to it. Secretion from the buccal glands and the duct of the parotid gland on a papilla opposite the fifth cheek tooth will drain into it.

33. (a) This fold is the sublingual frenulum which connects the ventral face of the tongue with the floor of the oral cavity at the sublingual recess.

(b) This structure is the sublingual caruncle of each side with the openings of the mandibular duct and the major sublingual duct, both of which conduct saliva from the mandibular and monostomatic sublingual salivary glands, respectively, to the oral cavity.

(c) Marker **C** is the upper lip or labia superior. This is composed of the m. obicularis oris and the m. levator nasolabialis (pars labialis).

(d) The muscles in (c) have a motor supply from the buccal branches of the facial (VII) nerve while the surface skin and lining mucosa derive sensation from the maxillary branch of the trigeminal (V) nerve.

(e) The tooth lying close to the marker is the third lower molar tooth. Lateral to it is the region of the buccal vestibule, the lateral boundary of which is formed by the m. buccinator.

34. (a) The markers are as follows: **Ai** — tongue, **Aii** — apex, **Aiii** — body and **Aiv** — root of tongue.

(b) Marker **Bi** shows the torus linguae while **Bii** shows the conical and lenticular papillae.

(c) Markers **C** show the cheek teeth or molars. These have a rough and serrated occlusal surface which results from continual wear during chewing. This surface consists of tissues of varying durability resulting in uneven wear which produces colour variation and an uneven folded pattern.

(d) The raised dorsum of the tongue and the torus linguae would suggest a ruminant, which is further supported by the lenticular and strong conical papillae.

(e) The bony structure is the ramus of the mandible. The m. masseter has been cut at **Eii**, while the m. pterygoideus has been cut at **Eiii**.

ANSWERS

35. (a) The regions are as follows: **Ai** — apex, **Aii** — body of tongue.
  (b) The structures are the vallate papillae.
  (c) Markers **C** show groups of foliate papillae.
  (d) Structures **D** are premolar and erupting molar teeth which are tuberculate (bunodont) in type. This type of cheek teeth is indicative of the porcine dentition and the tongue with its pointed apex and both vallate and foliate papillae support this conclusion.
  (e) Opening **Ei** is the aditus laryngis and **Eii** is the epiglottis.

36. (a) The markers are as follows: **Ai** — apex, **Aii** — body of tongue.
  (b) Markers **B** indicate the two vallate papillae.
  (c) Markers **C** show the regions of the foliate papillae. The horse tongue has a spatula appearance with a broad apex and a pair of vallate papillae with foliates.
  (d) Structures **D** are the cheek teeth. The rostral three are premolars while the caudal three are molars. These teeth are lophodont in type.
  (e) These structures are incisor teeth. The occlusal surface has a darkened hollow an infundibulum, which is present in all six teeth. The presence of all the molar teeth in wear would indicate that the animal had erupted all of its adult dentition. The presence of the infundibulum places the horse in the range of over four and half years but not yet over eight years of age.

37. (a) This prominence is the corniculate process of the arytenoid cartilage of the larynx.
  (b) Structure **B** is the dorsal border of the thyroid cartilage of the larynx. It articulates with the arytenoid cartilage, the cricoid cartilage and the thyrohoid bone.
  (c) **Ci** indicates the filiform papillae of the dorsum of the tongue which assist in holding the food on the tongue's surface. **Cii** is pointing to a cluster of foliate papillae which are situated at the dorsolateral border of the tongue. The latter are involved in the sense of taste.
  (d) This remnant is a portion of the mucous membrane of the floor of the oesophagus which lay dorsal to the larynx guarded at its entrance by the the fold of tissue called the limen pharyngoesophageum, shown at **Dii**.
  (e) The severed bony stump is the severed epihyoid bone, part of the hyoid apparatus which articulates with the skull at the mastoid process of the temporal bone.

38. (a) This bone is the second cervical vertebra (axis) of a dog.
  (b) This promontory is the dens (or odontoid process) which lies ventrally within the vertebral canal of the atlas. It is maintained in this position by the presence of the apical ligament of the dens which connects with the occipital bone by three strands or pillars and by the transverse atlantal ligament which runs transversely, dorsal to the dens, holding it ventrally against the ventral arch of the atlas. Rupture of the latter ligament causes the dens to come into contact dorsally with the spinal meninges and cord with possible severance of the cord causing quadraplegia and even death.
  (c) Surface **C** is the cranial articular surface of the axis (second cervical vertebra). It articulates with the caudal articular surface of the atlas (first cervical vertebra) and allows rotational movements of the head and atlas around a longitudinal axis. This is a pivot joint.
  (d) Aperture **D** is the transverse foramen which allows passage of the vertebral artery. and vein.
  (e) This is the spinous process of the axis which offers attachment to the predominantly elastic nuchal ligament. The spinous process is palpated subcutaneously in the dorsal midline immediately caudal to the external occipital protuberance.

39. (a) Area **A** is the intervertebral foramen through which passes the fourth spinal nerve — remember there are eight cervical spinal nerves. There will also be a cervical spinal arterial branch of the vertebral artery entering through the foramen.

(b) Area **B** is the intervertebral joint of the centra of cervical vertebrae 4 and 5. This joint space is occupied by the intervertebral disc in life.

(c) The darkened line is the joint space of the synovial joint between the articular processes of adjacent vertebrae 2 and 3.

(d) Bone **D** is the first thoracic vertebra. The bone bears the first truly elongated spinous process of the vertebral sequence. The seventh cervical vertebra has a small spinous process but this does not extend to a significant height dorsally. The first rib can be seen articulating with the body of the first thoracic vertebra.

(e) Structure **E** is the scapular spine. The other structure which it crosses over is the spinous process of the thoracic vertebra. Although the thickness of the scapular spine and the spinous process are similar the scapular spine lies along the plane of the direction of the rays of the X-ray beam. This produces a denser image compared with the flattened spinous process which lies at right angles to the beam.

40. (a) The region is the lateral projection of the cranial cervical region of a dog — the cranial region lies to the left. Bone **A** is the first cervical vertebra, the atlas.

(b) Area **B** represents the lateral vertebral foramen through which passes the vertebral artery.

(c) This shows the dorsal and ventral edges of the vertebral foramen or canal which allows conduction of the spinal cord with the three meningeal layers and vessels.

(d) Structure **D** is the transverse process of the atlas which can be readily palpated subcutaneously in a lateral position immediately caudal to the nuchal region of the skull.

(e) Structure **E** is the stylohoid bone which gives origin to the m. styloglossus, an extrinsic muscle of the tongue. Contraction of this muscle assists in retraction of the tongue if acting bilaterally or lateral deviation if acting unilaterally.

41. (a) Muscle **A** is the m. mylohoideus, which forms a muscular floor to the oral cavity. This muscle assists in elevating the cavity floor on contraction while pulling the hyoid apparatus cranially. The muscles meet at the median raphe and are innervated by the mandibular branch of the trigeminal (V) nerve.

(b) This is the mandibular salivary gland, the maxillary vein is seen laterally and the facial vein medially as it joins the lingual vein.

(c) This vessel is the external jugular vein which lies in a groove between the m. sternocephalicus medially and the m. brachiocephalicus laterally.

(d) Structure **D** is the ventral portion of the ring-like structure of the cricoid cartilage of the larynx. Attaching to it on each side is a rounded body of the m. cricothyroideus which is innervated by the cranial laryngeal nerve coming directly of the vagus (X) nerve. The other intrinsic muscles of the larynx receive innervation from the caudal laryngeal nerve which comes originally form the vagus (X) nerve but via the recurrent laryngeal nerve trunk.

(e) This structure is the carotid sheath containing the vagosympathetic trunk, the carotid artery and the internal jugular vein. The first contains the vagus (X) nerve running caudally and the sympathetic trunk running cranially, the second is running cranially while the third courses caudally.

ANSWERS

42. (a) Structure **A** is the mandibular lymph node which is responsible for drainage of the ventrorostral region of the head.

(b) This is the ventral laryngeal prominence of the thyroid cartilage of the larynx. It is formed by the union in midline of the two cartilaginous laminae of the thyroid cartilage.

(c) Structure **C** is the trachea which comprises a series of hyaline cartilage rings which are incomplete dorsally but bridged over by the smooth, transverse running, tracheal muscle. The adjacent rings are interconnected by the fibroelastic annular ligaments.

(d) Structure **D** is the longitudinally running oesophagus which commences at the pharynx and terminates at the cardia of the stomach in the left cranial abdomen. The wall comprises mainly layers of striated muscle in the dog.

(e) This is the m. longus coli which attaches to the bodies of adjacent cervical vertebrae but runs along the axial plane of the neck region. If the muscle is elevated from these attachments, the joints between the bodies of the cervical vertebrae are revealed with the intervertebral discs held *in situ* by the ventral longitudinal ligament. This is a surgical route used in the process of performing a disc fenestration.

43. (a) These are the arytenoid cartilages which are involved in the formation of the larynx.

(b) This is the m. cricoarytenoideus dorsalis which, on contraction, produces abduction of the vocal folds. It is innervated by the caudal laryngeal nerve which comes from the recurrent laryngeal nerve from the vagus (V) nerve.

(c) This tissue is the vocal fold which comprises the vocal ligament and the m. vocalis. It extends dorsally from the vocal process of the arytenoid cartilage to the ventral floor of the larynx which is formed by the thyroid cartilage.

(d) This space is the rima glottis, its width fluctuates during life as it is opened during inspiration by abduction of the vocal folds. The width can also fluctuate during sound production and will also narrow considerably if there is danger of foreign material passing through into the more caudal region of the laryngeal interior.

(e) The structures are as follows: **Ei** — the spinal cord, **Eii** — the dens (odontoid process) of the second cervical vertebra (axis) and **Eiii** — the body of the first cervical vertebra (atlas). The spinal cord lies in a vulnerable position with the dens immediately ventral to it as it protrudes over the body of the atlas. There is a transverse ligament of the atlas bridging dorsally over the dens to prevent damage being caused to the spinal cord.

44. (a) This vessel is the ascending aorta which arises from the left ventricle at the aortic valve.

(b) This vessel is the left common carotid artery which supplies oxygenated blood to head region including the brain. An alternative supply exists via the vertebral artery which can be seen running along the length of the cervical vertebrae, entering the transverse canal of the sixth cervical vertebra and running through the canal of each adjacent cervical vertebra.

(c) This is the axillary artery which is the major supplier of the thoracic limb. It arises from the subclavian artery and then passes cranially around the first rib to achieve the axillary space, to then follow on to the medial aspect of the brachium

(d) Vessel **D** is a coronary artery seen running on the surface of the heart, supplying oxygenated blood. The arteries arise from the aorta in the aortic bulb immediately distal to the aortic valve.

(e) Vessel **Ei** is the coeliac artery, supplying the stomach, proximal duodenum, liver and spleen while **Eii** is the cranial mesenteric artery which supplies the small intestine, caecum and proximal colon.

45. (a) Vessels **A** are the common carotid arteries which arise from the brachiocephalic trunk.
    (b) Vessels **B** are the vertebral arteries which arise from the subclavian arteries.
    (c) This is the basilar artery which contributes to the arterial circle of the brain, the circle of Willis.
    (d) This is the rostral cerebral artery.
    (e) The circle runs around the area of the dorsum sellae and surrounds the hypophysis cerebri (pituitary gland).

46. (a) The vessels are as follows: **Ai** — cranial vena cava, **Aii** — internal thoracic vein, **Aiii** — axillary vein, **Aiv** — costocervical veins.
    (b) This is the jugular vein, which drains the cranial region and also receives blood flow from the thoracic limb.
    (c) The vessels are as follows: **Ci** — linguofacial vein, **Cii** — maxillary vein. The mandibular and monostomatic sublingual salivary glands, within the same encapsulation, lie at the confluence of these veins.
    (d) Vessel **D** is a coronary vein which eventually drains into the right atrium at the coronary sinus.
    (e) Vessel **E** is the cephalic vein, which drains the thoracic limb of that side.

Thoracic Limb

47. (a) Area **A** is the brachium or arm region in which lies the humerus.
    (b) Region **B** is the antebrachium or forearm in which lie the radius and ulna. The marked aspect is cranial compared with the opposite aspect which is caudal.
    (c) This region is the manus or forepaw in which lie the bones of the carpus, the metacarpal bones and the phalanges. The aspect bearing the markers is dorsal compared with the opposite aspect which is palmar.
    (d) Region **D** is the carpal pad which lies immediately distal to the accessory carpal bone.
    (e) Region **E** is the point of the elbow — the olecranon process of ulna lies subcutaneously.

48. (a) This is the shoulder joint where the glenoid cavity of the scapula articulates with the head of the humerus.
    (b) This muscle is the m. brachiocephalicus (the m. cleidobrachialis portion of this muscle) which inserts onto the humerus, distal to its head. This acts as a protractor of the limb by extending the shoulder joint.
    (c) This is the elbow joint where the capitulum and the trochlea of the humerus articulate with the fovea of the radius and the trochlear notch of the ulna. These latter two bones also articulate with each other. The movements seen at the elbow joint are flexion and extension as well as limited supination and pronation.
    (d) The markers **Di** and **Dii** are indicating the first and fifth digits, respectively. The first consists of three major bones, a metacarpal and a proximal and a distal phalanx plus a proximal sesamoid. The fifth contains four major bones, a metacarpal and a proximal, middle and distal phalanx plus two proximal and one dorsal sesamoids.
    (e) This vessel is the cephalic vein which is used by clinicians for venepuncture (blood collection or drug administration). Running on either side of the vein at this point are the medial and lateral rami of the superficial branch of the radial nerve. Poor injection technique could result in erroneous deposition of irritant substances around the vein, involving the nerve trunks which results in severe irritation to the animal.

49. (a) This is the scapula from the left pectoral limb of an adult dog. The vertical scapular spine indicates the lateral aspect and the convex cranial border indicates a left scapula. The simple spine without any processes, except at the distal extremity, indicates a dog (cats have a suprahamate process directed caudally in distal third of scapular spine). Immature dogs under 12 months of age exhibit ongoing endochondral ossification with an active epiphyseal growth plate at the distal cranial point separating the supraglenoid process from the body of the scapula.

(b) Area **B** is the supraspinous fossa which is covered by the supraspinatus muscle in life.

(c) Structure **C** is the acromion process which gives attachment to the head of the deltoideus muscle.

(d) The deltoideus has another head of origin from the more proximal portion of the scapular spine. The two heads insert onto the deltoid tuberosity of the humerus. The muscle produces flexion of the shoulder joint.

(e) The axillary nerve provides the nerve supply. This is a mixed nerve from the brachial plexus, damage to which would result in loss of sensation over the caudolateral region of the shoulder joint region.

50. (a) This is the scapula; **Ai** shows the lateral aspect while **Aii** exhibits the medial surface.

(b) The structures are as follows: **Bi** — spinal tuberosity, **Bii** — the suprahamate process and **Biii** — the hamate process of the acromion. **Bii** indicates that this is the scapula of a cat.

(c) This region is the supraglenoid tubercle which gives origin to the m. biceps brachii which inserts onto the proximal radius.

(d) This region is the caudal border of scapula which gives origin to the m. teres major. The latter inserts onto the teres tuberosity on the medial aspect of the humerus.

(e) This is the facies serrata (serrated surface) of the scapula which gives attachment to the m. serratus ventralis. The latter also attaches to the transverse processes of the last five cervical vertebrae and the first seven or eight ribs.

51. (a) This is the lateral aspect of the scapula.

(b) The markers are as follows: **Bi** — caudal, **Bii** — cranial, **Biii** — dorsal border, **Biv** — ventral angle.

(c) The markers are as follows: **Ci** — spine of scapula, **Cii** — acromion process.

(d) This prominence is the supraglenoid process which gives origin to the m. biceps brachii.

(e) This is a bovine scapula which is triangular with a sinuous spine dividing the lateral surface unequally. The spine continues distally to terminate at a distinct acromion process (this would not occur in a horse).

52. (a) This is a scapula, the lateral surface is unevenly divided into a narrower supraspinous and a broader infraspinous fossa. The supraspinous fossa is always cranial which indicates a scapula from a left thoracic limb.

(b) This is the dorsal border. In the live animal this border is further enlarged by the presence of a cartilage plate which extends dorsally. As a normal consequence of the aging process this plate of cartilage can become calcified and then ossified which results in the irregular appearance.

(c) This is the scapular spine.

(d) This is the margin of glenoid cavity.

(e) This bone is an equine scapula. The bone is relatively narrow and the spine bears a distinct tuber halfway along the length of the scapula. There is no evidence of an acromion process at the distal end of the spine which is further indicative of the scapula of a horse.

53.(a) This a dog humerus. (i) The bone is relatively slender with a single intertubercular groove at the proximal end between the greater and lesser tubercles (c.f. double groove of horse). (ii) The greater tubercle is single (c.f. divided in horse) and at relatively the same height as the humeral head (c.f. elevated greater tubercle of ox and pig). (iii) An aperture, the supratrochlear foramen, is present at the distal end of the bone (c.f. larger species lack this aperture and the cat has a more lateral foramen, supracondylar foramen).

(b) The bone on the left displays the caudal aspect of the right humerus of a dog. The smooth contours of the articular surface of the proximally positioned humeral head face caudally. The deltoid tuberosity projecting from the right edge of the proximal shaft lies laterally. Both of these factors identify a right humerus.

(c) This is the tuberosity for the m. teres major. The m. latissimus dorsi also attaches here.

(d) This is the supratrochlear foramen. In the dog nothing passes directly through this opening.

(e) Area **E** is the capitulum of the humeral condyle which is in apposition with the fovea of the radius.

54.(a) Both bones are examples of the humerus. **Ai** is the left humerus as the greater tubercle, which is lateral in life, is lying to the right of this cranial view. **Aii** is the right humerus as this is a caudal view, as revealed by the full view of the head with the greater tubercle lying to the right.

(b) Each aperture is a supracondylar foramen. This type of opening at the distal end of the humerus, lying on the medial aspect, is characteristic of the cat. The dog has an aperture, the supratrochlear foramen, but it is placed in an axial position at the distal end of the humerus.

(c) The aperture allows passage of the brachial artery and the median nerve in the cat.

(d) This region is the trochlea of the condyle of humerus which articulates principally with the trochlear notch of the ulna.

(e) The region **Ei** is the tricipital line which gives origin to the lateral head of the m. triceps brachii. **Eii** is the deltoid tuberosity which receives the insertion of the m. deltoideus.

55.(a) This is a humerus.

(b) This is the head of the humerus.

(c) This region is the greater tuberosity.

(d) This is the deltoid tuberosity.

(e) This is an equine humerus — the double appearance of the greater tuberosity is indicative of a horse. The head is always directed caudally and the deltoid tuberosity laterally, this is thus a humerus from a left thoracic limb.

56.(a) This is the humerus.

(b) This is the greater tuberosity.

(c) This is the intertubercular groove.

(d) **Di** and **Dii** both lie on the condyle. **Di** specifically indicates the region of the capitulum, **Dii** indicates the trochlea.

(e) This is a bovine humerus. The greater tubercle lies laterally and the condylar surfaces are directed cranially, indicating the cranial face. The bone is therefore from a right thoracic limb. The greater tuberosity is massive, encroaching medially over the intertubercular groove. Both these observations support the answer.

ANSWERS

57. (a) This is the ventral angle of the scapula revealing its articular surface.

(b) This is the glenoid cavity. This is covered with articular cartilage and surrounded by a cartilaginous lip, the labrum glenoidale, which greatly increases the surface area for articulation.

(c) This is the supraglenoid tubercle which is directed cranially in the live animal.

(d) This is the acromion process which is directed laterally as it lies at distal end of the scapular spine.

(e) The tendons of insertion of the m. supraspinatus and m. infraspinatus lie in the area immediately lateral to the glenoid cavity.

58. (a) This is a view of the proximal extremity of the humerus.

(b) This marker identifies the humeral head which articulates with the glenoid cavity of the scapula in life.

(c) The projection is the lesser tubercle which lies on the medial surface of the humerus.

(d) The projection is the greater tubercle. The m. supraspinatus, the m. infraspinatus and the m. teres minor insert here.

(e) The depression is the intertubercular groove which has the tendon of origin of the m. biceps brachii, surrounded by the bicipital bursa, running over it in the live animal.

59. (a) This is a view of the distal extremity of the humerus.

(b) This area is the capitulum of the humeral condyle which articulates with the fovea of the proximal end of the radius.

(c) This area is the trochlea of the humeral condyle which articulates with the trochlear notch of the ulna.

(d) This area is the olecranon fossa which is found on the caudal aspect of the distal end of the humerus.

(e) The recess is associated with the anconeal process of the ulna.

60. (a) The line between **Ai** and **Aii** represents the articular line of the elbow joint which appears black as the surfaces are composed of cartilage with a small amount of joint fluid. The cartilage images as black on the radiograph. The line distal and cranial to **Aii** is also a cartilaginous line but it represents the growth plate of the proximal epiphysis of the radius and there is no joint fluid involved.

(b) This is the olecranon process of the ulna which is separated from the body by a growth plate for the proximal ulnar epiphysis. It normally images as a black line and should not be misinterpreted as a fracture.

(c) Bone **Ci** is a radius and **Cii** is an ulna. They are connected by an interosseus membrane and an interosseus ligament. Some degree of movement occurs between them during pronation and supination. They are restricted by the transversely placed annular ligament which runs from the ulna around the radial head in the region of the coronoid process.

(d) This is the proximal epiphysis of the humerus. The earliest secondary centre of ossification to appear radiographically is apparent as a small dot immediately after birth. It increases in size relative to the growth of the dog and will eventually fuse with the humeral body. This radiograph is of an immature pup as the growth plate is still open.

(e) This is the scapular region. The marker is lying in a position where the radiographic images of both scapulae are superimposed giving a dense image. Distally the image is less intense as there is no superimposition while cranial and proximally the air filled trachea is creating a less dense blacker image as it runs deep to the scapula.

61.(a) This is the shoulder joint which although spheroidal the movements are largely confined to the sagittal plane. This is brought about by flexion and extension of the joint (some abduction and adduction of the limb is possible but extremely limited).

(b) The angle of projection is a caudocranial projection — the lateral aspect lies to the right. This is verified by the scapular spine, acromion process and the greater tubercle of the proximal end of the humerus.

(c) There are poorly developed glenohumeral and coracohumeral ligaments. The major support comes from the tendons of insertion of the m. subscapularis medially and m. supraspinatus and m. infraspinatus laterally.

(d) The suprascapular nerve would travel here which passes cranially to the scapular neck and thus the shoulder joint when passing from medial to lateral. It is the motor nerve supply to the m. infraspinatus and the m. supraspinatus and so resulting loss of tone in these muscles following damage would affect the lateral support to the shoulder joint.

(e) This is the glenoid cavity. This is covered by hyaline cartilage in life but the overall dimension of the distal articular surface is much greater in the living animal due to the presence of an extending peripheral cartilage lip, the labrum glenoidale. Being cartilaginous, the lip is not imaged as part of the distal extremity of the scapula on the X-ray.

62.(a) The markers are as follows: **Ai** — neck, **Aii** — spine, **Aiii** — supraglenoid process of the scapula.

(b) The area is the glenoid cavity which articulates with the head of the humerus to form the shoulder joint.

(c) This is the greater tubercle of the humerus, which has two peaks. The scapula has a spine which fails to reach its distal region and lacks an acromion process. These features indicate a horse.

(d) This is the prominence of the deltoid tuberosity.

(e) The markers are as follows: **Ei** — body of first rib, **Eii** — manubrium sterni.

63.(a) This is the supracondylar foramen of the humerus.

(b) This aperture is only present in the cat. The clavicles are also indicative of this species as they are seen bilaterally as thin white lines immediately cranial to the shoulder joint.

(c) The median nerve and brachial artery pass through the foramen in the cat.

(d) These bony shafts are the radius and ulna. The ulnar shaft, or body, is the most lateral of the two in the distal portion of the forearm.

(e) The apparently separate element is the epiphyseal growth plate of the ulna which will develop into the fused styloid process of the adult ulna. This is a normal feature of the immature cat.

64.(a) This is the m. trapezius which is a protractor and abductor of the limb. The nerve supply is the accessory nerve.

(b) This muscle is the m. triceps, long head, which is the flexor of the shoulder and extensor of the elbow. The nerve supply is the radial nerve.

(c) This is the m. cleidobrachialis (part of the m. brachiocephalicus) which is the protractor of the limb and extensor of the shoulder. Unilaterally, it turns the head to one side or bilaterally lowers the head by flexion of the cervical region. This head of the m. brachiocephalicus is innervated by the axillary nerve. The main components of the muscle receive innervation from the accessory nerve and ventral rami of the cervical spinal nerves.

(d) This muscle is the m. cutaneous trunci. This muscle is responsible for skin movements over the lateral thoracic and abdominal region, its motor supply is by the lateral thoracic nerve.

(e) The muscle **A** would not be affected as the accessory nerve is derived from cranial nerve sources. Muscle **B** would lose its motor function as the radial nerve is derived from the brachial plexus nerve sources. Muscle **C** would lose some motor function to this component as the axillary nerve is derived from the brachial plexus, but the overall muscle would still receive motor input from the accessory nerve and cervical ventral spinal nerves which are given off the cranial to brachial plexus. Muscle **D** would lose motor input as the lateral thoracic nerve is derived from brachial plexus sources.

65. (a) This is the m. teres minor which produces flexion of shoulder joint. It overlies the caudolateral aspect of the shoulder joint capsule.

(b) This is the m. triceps brachii which produces flexion of the shoulder joint and extension of the elbow joint.

(c) This is the m. brachialis which produces flexion of the elbow joint.

(d) This is the m. extensor carpi radialis which produces extension of the carpus.

(e) This is the radial nerve. Lesions of the radial nerve at this level would affect only the m. extensor carpi radialis (**D**) but the m. triceps brachii (**B**), although supplied by the radial nerve, would escape paralysis as the motor supply has been given off more proximally. The m. teres minor (**A**) would be unaffected because its motor supply is from the axillary nerve as would the m. brachialis (**C**) with its motor supply from the musculocutaneous nerve.

66. (a) This is the medial aspect of the shoulder and brachium. **Ai** is the m. latissimus dorsi, **Aii** is the m. trapezius, **Aiii** is the m. serratus ventralis, **Aiv** is the m. cleidobrachialis (m. brachiocephalicus) and **Av** is the mm. pectorales superficiales and profundus.

(b) This is the m. teres major which arises from the caudal scapular border and inserts onto the tuberosity of the teres major on the medial aspect of the humerus. The m. teres major causes flexion of the shoulder joint.

(c) This is the m. supraspinatus which arises from the supraspinous fossa of the lateral aspect of the scapula and inserts onto the greater tubercle of the humerus. This muscle extends the shoulder joint and offers collateral support to that joint.

(d) This is the m. biceps brachii which arises from the supraglenoid tubercle and inserts onto the proximal radius. This muscle primarily flexes the elbow joint but is secondary extensor of shoulder joint.

(e) The nerves are as follows: **Ei** — suprascapular nerve, **Eii** — axillary nerve and **Eiii** — musculocutaneous nerve. **Ei** innervates muscle **C**, **Eii** innervates muscle **B** and **Eiii** innervates muscle **D**.

67. (a) The bone is the radius. **Ai** is the cranial aspect, **Aii** is the caudal aspect.

(b) The markers are as follows: **Bi** — fovea, which articulates with the capitulum of the humerus. **Bii** — trochlea or carpal articular surface, which meets with the radial carpal bone in the carpal joint.

(c) This is the radial tuberosity where the m. biceps brachii inserts.

(d) This is the styloid process which lies on the medial surface of the radius.

(e) This is the nutrient foramen which allows access to a nutrient artery, permitting it to penetrate through to the medullary cavity and the endosteal layer.

68.(a) **A** is the anconeal process of the ulna of a dog. The ulna is fully formed throughout its length eliminating ox and horse. The pig ulna would be more massive distally and the cat has a more cranially directed proximal extremity (olecranon process). Structure **A** lies within the olecranon fossa of the humerus in the standing dog.

(b) This is the coronoid process which articulates with the articular circumference of the proximal radius.

(c) This is the olecranon process which receives tendon of insertion of the m. triceps brachii.

(d) This is the styloid process of the ulna which articulates with the distal articular surface of the radius at the ulnar notch, ulnar carpal bone and accessory carpal bone.

(e) Structures **B**, **C** and **D** are all palpable but **A** is within the olecranon fossa except at times of maximum flexion of the elbow joint.

69.(a) These bones are the radius and ulna.

(b) This is the olecranon of the ulna.

(c) This region is the anconeal process of the ulna. The process is housed within the olecranon fossa of the humerus in the extended elbow joint.

(d) This region is the styloid process of the ulna.

(e) These are the radius and ulna of a cow. The ulna is represented distally but is fused to the radius throughout its length. The pig would have a separate radius and ulna and the horse an imperfectly formed distal ulna. The styloid process of the ulna is located laterally and the olecranon caudally. The bones are therefore from the right thoracic limb.

70.(a) These bones are the radius and ulna.

(b) This is the trochlear notch of the ulna.

(c) This is the radial tuberosity onto which attaches the tendon of the m. biceps brachii.

(d) This is the lateral styloid process which appears to be part of the radius.

(e) This is the radius and ulna of a horse. The ulna appears to be incomplete distally and is fusing with the radius proximally, characteristic of this species. The position of the ulna lying caudally and the lateral styloid process indicate that these bones are from the left thoracic limb. In the horse the lateral styloid process is all that remains of the distal epiphysis of the ulna but it appears fused to, and thus looks like part of, the radius. It is, however, developmentally part of the ulna.

71.(a) This is the craniocaudal view of the elbow joint of a dog.

(b) This represents the joint space of the elbow between humerus and the radius and ulna. The joint surfaces are cartilaginous, lacking radiodensity, giving the dark appearance.

(c) This represents the proximal radio-ulnar joint, the joint space and cartilaginous articular surfaces image as a dark line. The joint can carry out pronation and supination to a limited extent, being produced by contraction of the m. pronator teres and the m. supinator.

(d) This is the olecranon process of the ulna seen superimposed over the distal humerus.

(e) Markers **Ei** and **Eii** are, respectively, the lateral and medial epicondyles of the humerus. Proximally the ulna lies in a caudomedial position articulating with the narrower portion of the humeral condyle, the trochlea, which lies medially.

ANSWERS

72.(a) This is the carpal region and manus of the right thoracic limb of a horse. The caudal and palmar aspects are visible.

(b) The horse is an unguligrade animal as it walks on an upright digit and protects its distal digit with a horny hoof. It has only one weight bearing digit, the third digit, and as this is an odd number it falls into the category of being a perissodactyla.

(c) The markers are as follows: Ci — distal phalanx, Cii — palmar processes. The ungual cartilages attach to these structures.

(d) This region is the carpal canal which is formed by the flexor retinaculum (transverse ligament of the carpus) bridging over from the accessory carpal bone laterally to the medial aspect of the joint. The tendons of the superficial and deep digital flexor muscles pass through the canal.

(e) The areas are as follows: Ei — proximal scutum, Eii — middle scutum, Eiii — distal scutum. The tendons of the superficial and deep digital flexor tendons run over Ei; the deep digital flexor tendon runs over Eii and Eiii. The tendons are held by annular ligaments. The tendons are held in place at Ei by the superficial transverse metacarpal ligament (palmar annular ligament) and at Eii and Eii by the proximal and distal digital annular ligaments.

73.(a) This is the carpal joint of a horse. Marker A is overlying the radial carpal bone.

(b) This bone is the intermediate carpal bone.

(c) This is the ulnar carpal bone.

(d) The markers outline the accessory carpal bone.

(e) This is the first carpal bone which has been imaged superimposed upon the second carpal bone. The marker for the first carpal bone lies medially as the accessory carpal bone lies laterally.

74.(a) This is the olecranon process. The portion of bone appears to be separated from the body of the ulna but the dark line represents a line of cartilage, the epiphyseal growth plate which is radiolucent. Thus, the proximal epiphysis for the olecranon is attached to the ulnar body in life by cartilage in the immature dog and by bone in the adult dog.

(b) This is the supratrochlear foramen of the distal end of the humerus. This is imaged in almost all dog limbs at all ages except in a few of the smaller shorter legged breeds such as the Cairn or Aberdeenshire Terrier where the foramen is closed over by a thin plate of bone.

(c) This represents the epiphyseal growth cartilage separating the centre of ossification of the medial humeral epicondyle from the ossifying body of the humerus. This is constant in all immature dogs but the growth cartilage will be replaced at the time of maturity by ossified material which will image as a white line in the adult dog.

(d) This is the centre of ossification for the distal extremity of the metacarpal bone — part of the proximal bone. The distal bone, proximal phalanx, also has a secondary centre of ossification which is situated at its proximal extremity. This is imaged as a smaller flatter structure at the proximal end of the body of the proximal phalanx, just distal to structure D.

(e) The darker line represents the joint space of the proximal interphalangeal joint of the first digit. The joint surfaces, being cartilaginous, image as black and as they are superimposed over the body of another metacarpal bone they give the erroneous impression of a fracture. Its appearance is always dependent on the angle at which the manus is X-rayed and is therefore variable. The first digit is often removed within a few days of birth and so the first digit would frequently be absent on X-rays of dog limbs.

75. (a) This is the growth plate of the distal epiphysis of an equine third metacarpal bone.
(b) This is the joint space of a metacarpophalangeal (fetlock) joint.
(c) This is the growth plate of the only epiphysis of the proximal phalanx.
(d) This is the joint space of the proximal interphalangeal (pastern) joint.
(e) This is the growth plate of the only epiphysis of the middle phalanx. **A, C** and **E** appear dark as they consist of cartilaginous plates which allow longitudinal growth to take place. **B** and **D** are dark as they represent lines of opposed layers of hyaline cartilage but in these cases narrow joint spaces are also present with synovial fluid in the joint space.

76. (a) This is the lateral epicondyle of the humerus which gives attachment to the lateral collateral ligament of the elbow joint.
(b) This is the m. extensor digitorum communis which extends the carpus and digits; it is innervated by the radial nerve.
(c) The is the m. flexor carpi ulnaris (ulnar head) which flexes the carpus; it is innervated by the ulnar nerve.
(d) If the nerve (radial) to muscle **B** was severed there would be loss of sensation over the dorsum of the antebrachium and digits except for the most lateral border of the fifth digit. Severance of the nerve (ulnar) to **C** would result in loss of cutaneous sensation of the palmolateral aspect of distal antebrachium and manus, including the most dorsolateral border of fifth digit.
(e) This vessel is the cephalic vein which carries blood form the manus distally to the proximal brachium where the blood can either flow directly or via the omobrachial vein to join the jugular vein. Alternatively, it can pass through the axillo-brachial vein to join the brachial vein and thus the subclavian to the brachiocephalic vein.

77. (a) This is the medial aspect of the antebrachium (forearm) of a dog. The marker itself is indicating the m. triceps brachii.
(b) This muscle is the m. flexor digitorum superficialis.
(c) This muscle is the m. flexor carpi radialis.
(d) This feature is the medial epicondyle of the humerus, a palpable landmark in the dog. A general rule is that the flexor muscles of the distal limb originate from the medial epicondyle and so muscle **B** flexes the carpus and digits while muscle **C** flexes the carpus.
(e) This is the median nerve which is responsible for muscles **B** and **C**. Muscle **A** is innervated by the radial nerve.

78. (a) This is the left thoracic limb. The accessory carpal bone lies laterally in the carpal region and the first digit lies medially in the manus.
(b) This is the m. extensor carpi ulnaris. Although it is innervated by the radial nerve and has its origins on the lateral epicondyle (as is the common rule for extensors of the carpus and digits) its insertion onto the accessory carpal bone is at such an angle that it can appear to act as a flexor when the limb is at certain postural angles. It is often termed the m. ulnaris lateralis to avoid confusion between its name and its function.
(c) This is the m. flexor digitorum superficialis. This is a digit flexor, innervated by the median nerve.
(d) These are the tendons of insertion of the superficial digital flexor which run to insert onto the proximal palmar surface of the middle phalanges. They form a sleeve-like structure (manica) to permit the tendon of the deep digital flexor to pass distally to insert onto the distal phalanx.

(e) This is the digital pad which acts as a protective layer/frictional device due to the hyperkeratinised papillated stratified squamous epithelial layer overlying the elastic reticulum with an intermingling adiposa. The structures lying deep to it, and thus vulnerable in the case of deep cuts, are the distal interphalangeal joint and tendon of the deep digital flexor muscle. Complete section of the deep flexor tendon would cause dorsal hyperextension of the toe due to the pull of the dorsal elastic ligament and loss of ability to counteract the dorsal pull due to a failure to flex the distal interphalangeal joint.

79. (a) This is the carpal joint and manus of a dog. **Ai** is the dorsal view and **Aii** is the palmar view.

(b) The bones are as follows: **Bi** — radial, **Bii** — ulnar, **Biii** — accessory carpal bones. The radial bone is originally derived from centres of ossification for the radial and intermediate carpal bones but they fuse to form what is termed the radial carpal bone. The ulnar arises from a single centre. The accessory has a centre for body and a secondary centre for the palmar extremity.

(c) The bones are as follows: **Ci** — first, **Cii** — second, **Ciii** — third and **Civ** — fourth carpal bones. **Ci** is the most medial and **Civ** the most lateral bone.

(d) These bones are the dorsal sesamoids which are retained in their position dorsal to the metacarpophalangeal joint by being intercalated into the tendon of insertion for each digit (except the first digit) of the m. extensor digitorum communis.

(e) The markers are indicating the pairs of proximal sesamoid bones. The palmar (intersesamoidean) ligament runs between these bones while the tendons of the mm. flexor digitorum superficialis and profundus course over them. These tendons are held in position by the palmar annular ligament (superficial transverse metacarpal ligament).

80. (a) **Ai** is the metacarpal bone and line **Aii** indicates the location of a groove on its dorsal aspect. This bone, although apparently having a single body, is derived from the fusion of two metacarpal bones. This line indicates the line of fusion.

(b) This is a pair of proximal sesamoid bones. The presence of two pairs of such bones and dual origin of the metacarpal bone with divided distal articular surfaces indicates a ruminant and the overall size suggests a bovine manus.

(c) This is the distal sesamoid bone.

(d) The markers are as follows: **Di** — distal phalanx, **Dii** — extensor process.

(e) The marker is pointing to an area on the axial border of the hoof where the hard keratinised wall suddenly merges with the softer horn of the bulb of heel giving an area vulnerable to penetration by foreign bodies. This area is referred to as the axial or paraconal groove.

81. (a) These bones are as follows: **Ai** — third metacarpal, **Aii** — fourth metacarpal, **Aiii** — second metacarpal of a horse.

(b) These structures are the proximal sesamoids which are connected by the palmar (intersesamoidean) ligament. This forms the proximal scutum for the passage of the flexor tendons of digit.

(c) This prominence is the sagittal ridge of the distal extremity of the third metacarpal which lies in the metacarpophalangeal joint space. It interlocks with a corresponding groove in the articular surface of the proximal phalanx and assists in limiting movement of the joint to flexion and extension.

(d) The lines forming a V-shaped impression are created by a roughened surface for the attachment of the oblique sesamoidean ligament on the palmar aspects of the proximal phalanx.

(e) This darkened area is created by the nutrient foramen, a deficiency in the cortical bone to permit transfer of a blood vessel. This is a normal feature of a long bone.

82. (a) This is the proximal interphalangeal joint space of a horse. The proximal phalanx lies proximally and the middle phalanx distally.

(b) This is the distal sesamoid (navicular) bone which is held in apposition to the middle and distal phalanges by the presence of the tendon of the deep digital flexor on its palmar surface. It also has collateral ligaments which run from the proximal phalanx to the sesamoid bone and a single unpaired sheet, the distal ligament, which runs between the sesamoid bone and the flexor surface of the distal phalanx.

(c) This is the distal interphalangeal joint which permits flexion and extension, although some degree of rotation is possible to permit the horse to cope with maintaining ground contact on uneven surfaces.

(d) The markers are as follows: **Di** — extensor process, **Dii** — semilunar canal of the distal phalanx.

(e) This image represents a nail holding the shoe in place. In correct shoeing the nail should be placed in the horn of the wall, peripheral to the white line. This is a forelimb as the overall shape is evenly cresentic, the hindlimb would be narrower and more oval in outline. Furthermore, there is only a single toe clip placed at the point of toe (the hindlimb is usually shod with two clips, one placed in each quarter of the wall).

83. (a) These are the solar surfaces of the hooves of a horse. **Ai** is evenly cresentic in outline, indicating a thoracic limb. **Aii** is narrower and more oval in outline, indicating a pelvic limb.

(b) The markers are as follows: **Bi** — frog, **Bii** — central sulcus, **Biii** — lateral sulcus of the frog.

(c) The markers are as follows: **Ci** — wall at the toe, **Cii** — wall at the quarters, **Ciii** — angle, **Civ** — bars of hoof.

(d) This is the sole. The white line demarcates the wall from the sole in the live animal. The region peripheral to the white line is insensitive but the area within the white line is sensitive. It is used as the demarcating line for introduction of nails during shoeing.

(e) When the hoof hits the ground the frog should impact first to absorb concussive forces. The wall at the periphery of the hoof should bear the weight on the ground surface in the normal standing horse.

84. (a) The structures are as follows: **Ai** — tendon of the m. flexor digitalis superficialis, **Aii** — tendon of the m. flexor digitalis profundus, **Aiii** — the accessory ligament (inferior check ligament) of the deep flexor tendon, **Aiv** — m. interosseus (suspensory ligament).

(b) This is the joint space of the metacarpophalangeal joint (fetlock). The third metacarpal bone and the proximal phalanx are found on the dorsal aspect, while the two proximal sesamoid bones are found on the palmar aspect.

(c) This structure is the complimentary cartilage of the middle phalanx onto which inserts the straight sesamoidean ligament. The tendon of the superficial digital flexor also inserts here.

(d) This is the distal sesamoid (navicular) bone. The middle and distal phalanges can be found on the dorsal suface of this bone and the tendon of the m. flexor digitalis profundus can be found on its palmar surface.

(e) This is the digital cushion which contains a feltwork of reticular fibres, collagen, adipose tissue and blood vessels; this structure is anticoncussive in function. The species is the horse.

85. (a) This is the tendon of the m. flexor digitalis superioris which terminates by forming a sleeve-like structure, a manica, which allows the tendon of the deep flexor to penetrate though it. The superficial tendon eventually inserts onto the distal tubercles of the proximal phalanx and the complimentary cartilage of the middle phalanx at the level of the proximal interphalangeal joint.

(b) This is the tendon of the m. flexor digitalis profundus which terminates on the flexor face of the distal phalanx after passing over the palmar surface of the distal sesamoid (navicular) bone.

(c) This is the accessory ligament (inferior check ligament) of the deep flexor tendon. This ligament merges into the deep surface of the deep flexor tendon.

(d) This is the m. interosseus or suspensory ligament. This ligament runs onto the abaxial surfaces of the proximal sesamoid bones before coursing onto the dorsal surface to eventually merge with the tendon of the m. extensor digitalis communis.

(e) This space is the synovial sheath of the deep digital flexor, in life it contains synovial fluid.

86. (a) This prominence is the styloid process of the radius of a dog.

(b) This is the accessory carpal bone which lies at right angles to the long axis of the limb. Thus, on a dorsopalmar projection of the radiograph this bone is imaged in the long axis providing a denser radiographic image.

(c) This is the fourth carpal bone.

(d) These are the proximal sesamoid bones (palmar). A cartilaginous intersesamoidean ligament connects pairs of sesamoids and runs between adjacent pairs. Over this connecting cartilaginous channel run the tendons of the superficial and deep flexors of the digits held down by an annular ligament.

(e) This is the ungual crest of the distal phalanx which is the area of attachment of the corium of the claw.

87. (a) This vessel is the brachial artery which arises from the axillary artery.

(b) Vessel **B** is the radial artery.

(c) Vessel **Ci** is the median artery which can be seen giving off the common interosseus artery at **Cii**.

(d) Vessel **Di** is a palmar common digital artery while the lesser vessel **Dii** is a palmar metacarpal artery.

(e) Vessel **E** is the palmar proper digital artery which lies on the palmar aspect of the digit on the side closest to the axial line of the manus.

88. (a) This vessel is the cephalic vein which eventually flows into the jugular vein.

(b) This is the median cubital vein which interconnects the cephalic with the median vein.

(c) This is the brachial vein which flows into the axillary vein.

(d) This is the internal thoracic vein which is situated on the ventral floor of the thoracic cavity.

(e) The clinician would chose the cephalic vein (**A**) which is conveniently found subcutaneously on the cranial surface, in the proximal antebrachial region.

Thorax

89. (a) These are thirteen thoracic vertebrae of a dog; the first (most cranial) vertebra lies to the left.

(b) These are the spinous processes which give origin to the m. trapezius and the m. rhomboideus. The former inserts onto the proximal scapular spine, and the latter onto the medial aspect of the dorsal border of the scapula.

(c) This is the anticlinal eleventh thoracic vertebra which bears a nearly perpendicular spinous process (all succeeding spinous processes are directed cranially). It therefore represents the transition segment of the thoracolumbar region.

(d) The areas **Di** and **Dii** are the cranial and caudal costal foveas, respectively. These articulate with the heads of the ribs and form synovial joints between the ribs and the vertebrae.

(e) This is the mamillary process which projects from the dorsal surface of the transverse process.

90. (a) Bone **A** is the seventh cervical vertebra as the first rib can be seen immediately caudal to it.

(b) Bone **B** is the twelfth thoracic vertebra as it is the next adjacent vertebra to the eleventh vertebra which has a near perpendicular spinous process while the twelfth has a cranially directed spinous process.

(c) Bone **C** is the first lumbar vertebra as it does not have articulations with a rib.

(d) This aperture is the intervertebral foramen through which emerges a spinal nerve in life.

(e) The bones are as follows: **Ei** — first rib, **Eii** — twelfth rib, **Eiii** — thirteenth rib. **Ei** articulates with the sternum, **Eii** unites with the cartilage of ribs ten and eleven to form the costal arch while **Eiii** has its distal end floating free in the musculature of the lateral wall.

91. (a) This is the m. omotransversarius which originates from the wing of atlas, inserts onto the distal scapular spine and protracts the limb.

(b) This is the m. trapezius which originates from the mid-dorsal raphe of the cervical region and the third to the ninth thoracic vertebrae. It inserts onto the scapular spine. This muscle elevates and protracts the limb.

(c) This is the m. latissimus dorsi which originates through the lumbodorsal fascia from the last seven thoracic vertebrae and the lumbar vertebrae. It produces retraction of the limb and flexion of the shoulder joint, and when the limb is fixed it draws the trunk forward.

(d) This is the m. pectoralis profundus which originates from the sternum and inserts onto the lesser tubercle of the humerus with an aponeurosis extending over the m. biceps brachii to the greater tubercle. This muscle retracts the limb or produces extension of the shoulder joint depending on the relative position of the limb. Its position causes it to draw the limb towards the trunk.

(e) If the bracial plexus was totally damaged **A** and **B** would be unaffected as they receive their nerve supply from the accessory (XI) nerve which does not come through the plexus. **C** and **D** would be affected as the thoracodorsal and pectoral nerves are formed through the brachial plexus.

92. (a) This is the m. scalenus which acts to pull the neck downwards or unilaterally to pull the neck to the side. This muscle assists in inspiration if the neck is fixed.

ANSWERS

(b) This is the m. serratus ventralis which originates from the transverse processes of the last five cervical vertebrae and the first eight ribs. This produces both protraction and retraction of the thoracic limb and, when the limb is fixed, assists in inspiration.

(c) This is the m. splenius which lies on the lateral cervical region. This extends and raises the head and neck or unilaterally draws the head and neck laterally.

(d) An incision would pass through the mm. intercostales externi and interni, endothoracic fascia and parietal pleura. If continued more ventrally the incision would involve the m. obliquus externus abdominis.

(e) This muscle group is the mm. pectorales which inserts onto the proximal humerus. It is innervated by the pectoral nerves from the brachial plexus.

93. (a) This is the trachea which extends throughout the cranial thorax and terminates at the level of the fifth thoracic vertebra by bifurcating into the left and right principal bronchi. It would, therefore, not be seen in cross-section caudal to this level.

(b) This is the aorta which conveys blood from the left ventricle to the systemic circulation. This vessel has a relatively thick wall, high in elastic tissue.

(c) This is the oesophagus which runs from the thoracic inlet to exit from the thorax via the hiatus oesophageus in the diaphragm. It would, therefore, be seen in cross-section throughout the length of the thorax.

(d) This is the heart which is covered by the epicardium and the pericardium within the mediastinum.

(e) This is the left auricle cut in cross-section. It is lying on the same side of the thorax as the aorta which is a left-sided structure.

94. (a) This is the tendinous centre of the diaphragm. This attaches to the ventral surfaces of the lumbar vertebrae, the ribs and sternum.

(b) The markers are as follows: **Bi** — cranial part of cranial lobe, **Bii** — caudal part of cranial lobe, **Biii** — caudal lobe of the left lung.

(c) This is the heart. This is overlaid by the mediastinum, parietal pericardium and visceral pericardium (epicardium).

(d) This is a portion of thymus, lying ventrally in the mediastinal space. This organ varies considerably in size depending on the age of the dog. In a young dog, as shown, the organ is extensive and occupies most of the ventral cranial mediastinal area. In an aged dog, the organ regresses and is then seen as a small vestigial structure occupying a much reduced area of mediastinal space.

(e) This is the brachial plexus. The nerves contributing to the plexus are the ventral branches of the fifth to eighth cervical spinal nerves and the first, and possibly the second, thoracic spinal nerves. These nerves emerge from the vertebral canal via the intervertebral foramina.

95. (a) The markers are as follows: **Ai** — pars costali, **Aii** — pars sternalis of diaphragm. This is the major muscle responsible for inspiration; it is innervated by the phrenic nerve which comes from the ventral branches of cervical nerves five, six and seven.

(b) This space is the right costodiaphragmatic recess. It is formed laterally by the thoracic wall, comprised of ribs and the mm. intercostales, and medially by the diaphragm. The former is covered by the serous membrane of the parietal pleura and the latter by the diaphragmatic pleura.

(c) The markers are as follows: **Ci** — cranial lobe, **Cii** — middle lobe and **Ciii** — caudal lobe of the right lung.

(d) The space created here between the cranial and middle lung lobes is the cardiac notch. The space reveals the heart.

(e) These structures are the intercostal artery, vein and nerve which are located caudal to the rib in a groove. This is an important factor to remember when making intercostal incisions, by trying to avoid incising too close to the caudal edge. The intercostal artery arises from the dorsal aorta and anastomoses with the arterial supply coming ventrally from the internal thoracic artery. The venous drainage runs either ventrally into the internal thoracic vein or dorsally, eventually to the vena azygos.

96. (a) This is the left lung.

(b) The markers are as follows: **Bi** — cranial lobe, **Bii** — middle lobe, **Biii** — caudal lobe of lung.

(c) The markers are as follows: **Ci** — larynx, **Cii** — trachea.

(d) This is the oesophagus.

(e) The trachea is short and the larynx has a double corniculate process of the arytenoid cartilage. The right lung has an undivided cranial lobe and a middle lobe while the left lung has a divided cranial lobe. There is evidence of lobulation on the lung surface. All these factors suggest a porcine lung.

97. (a) This is the heart. Ai is the right ventricle which lies in this far cranial position, **Aii** is the left auricle, which lies more dorsally nearer the heart base. **Aiii** is the left ventricle, which lies closer to the caudoventrally directed apex of the heart.

(b) This is the dorsal aorta which arises firstly from the left ventricle, then the aortic arch. It exits the thorax by passing through the diaphragm at the hiatus aorticus in the dorsal region of the thorax between the diaphragmatic crura.

(c) This is the thymus which lies in the cranial mediastinal space.

(d) These vessels are the internal thoracic artery and vein which serve the structures found around the ventral floor of the thorax and cranial abdomen, being continued caudally as cranial epigastric vessels.

(e) This is the accessory lobe of the right lung which lies in the serous fold of the plica vena cava. This fold also bears the right phrenic nerve and the caudal vena cava.

98. (a) This is the foramen venae cavae which is found in the region of the centrum tendineum of the diaphragm. This permits passage of the caudal vena cava from the abdominal to the thoracic cavity.

(b) This is the cranial vena cava which terminates in the right atrium of the heart. This receives contributories from the right azygos and right costocervical veins. These vessels drain the dorsal thoracic wall while the former also receives blood from the broncho-oesophageal vein.

(c) This strand is the phrenic nerve which originates from the ventral branches of the fifth, sixth, seventh and eighth cervical nerves. It terminates on the diaphragm which it supplies, arriving at this muscle with the caudal vena cava.

(d) This is the oesophagus. The vagus nerve is indicated running along its surface which enters the thorax at the thoracic inlet as the vagosympathetic trunk. This exits the thorax via the hiatus oesophageus along with the oesophagus.

(e) The markers are as follows: **Ei** — the right atrium, **Eii** — the right ventricle. Separating the two markers is the region of the coronary groove which here contains the right coronary artery.

ANSWERS

99. (a) This is the vagus nerve which courses along the oesophagus to exit caudally from the thorax at the hiatus oesophageus with the oesophagus.

(b) This is the dorsal aorta which exits caudally from the thorax at the hiatus aorticus between the crura of the diaphragm where it is accompanied by the thoracic duct.

(c) This is the sympathetic trunk which runs from the thorax into the abdomen by passing through the gap between the dorsal lumbar origins and the lateral costal origins of the diaphragm. It is bridged over by the lumbar musculature dorsally and the diaphragm ventrally.

(d) This is the caudal vena cava which passes from the abdomen to the thorax via the foramen venae cavae.

(e) This is the xiphoid process of the sternum.

100. (a) Marker **Ai** is indicating the position of the heart with the trachea (**Aii**) lying dorsal to its base. The trachea bifurcates at this level.

(b) Marker **Bi** is indicating the position of the liver with the gall bladder (**Bii**) lying between the liver lobes.

(c) This is a sectioned portion of stomach.

(d) This is the distended urinary bladder which reaches cranially to the umbilical region; an empty bladder would be found more caudally near the pelvic inlet.

(e) This is the rectum which lies in the pelvic cavity with the sacral vertebrae dorsally and the pelvic symphysis of the pubis and ischium lying ventrally.

101. (a) This is the aorta which runs from the left ventricle of the heart to the hiatus aorticus in the dorsal diaphragm.

(b) This is the caudal vena cava which runs from the foramen venae cavae to the right atrium of heart.

(c) This is the trachea which runs from the thoracic inlet to bifurcate dorsally to the cranial part of the base of the heart .

(d) These are the dorsal bronchi running through the caudal lobe of the lung.

(e) This is the right ventricle of the heart which is situated cranioventrally relative to the outline of the heart.

102. (a) This is the apex of the heart.

(b) This is the base of the heart.

(c) This represents the gas which has accumulated within the fundus of the stomach.

(d) This is the diaphragm with liver lying deep to it. The diaphragm alone is only a thin muscular layer but the liver produces a more dense radio-opaque image.

(e) The marker lies on the left side. (a) and (c) assist in proving the point as the apex of the heart lies to the left and the fundus of the stomach is found on the left-hand side of the midline.

103. (a) This is the foramen venae cavae, where the caudal vena cava passes from an abdominal position (dorsal to the liver) to run through the diaphragm and thus into the caudal mediastinal space of the thoracic cavity.

(b) A penetrating needle would pass through the skin, the m. cutaneous trunci, the costal origins of the m. obliquus abdominis externus, the mm. intercostales, the endothoracic fascia, the parietal pleura and the left ventricular wall, to finally locate in the lumen of the left ventricle.

(c) This is the maxilla of the skull.

(d) This is the frontal sinus.

(e) This is the clavicle which is found as a consistent bony structure in cats. The shortened maxillary area shown at **A**, resulting in the reduced length of the facial region and the pronounced frontal profile of **B**, also assists in identifying the species.

104. (a) This is the cross-section of the heart made at a level ventral to the coronary groove.
(b) The markers are as follows: **Bi** — right ventricle (thinner free wall), **Bii** — left ventricle (thicker free wall).
(c) Both ventricles contain the same volume of blood but the right ventricle contains deoxygenated blood and the left contains oxygenated blood.
(d) This is the interventricular septum.
(e) These are the papillary muscles which have the chordae tendineae attached to them in life.

105. (a) This is the right ventricle through which flows deoxygenated blood. The right ventricular free wall is much thinner than that of the left ventricle.
(b) This is the left atrioventricular (mitral) valve which divides the left atrium from the left ventricle by means of valvular flaps with serrated edges.
(c) Theses are the chordae tendineae which stretch from the papillary muscles on the ventricular wall to the serrated edges of the atrioventricular valve flaps. These assist in preventing the valve flaps from being pushed back into the atrium.
(d) This is the aortic valve, which consists of three semilunar cusps which separate the left ventricular outflow tract from the aorta. This forms a barrier as the cusps are floated into a closed position by retrograde eddying currents in the aortic sinuses.
(e) This is the coronary vein cut in cross-section. This conveys deoxygenated blood back from the myocardium to the coronary sinus of the right atrium.

106. (a) This is the left ventricle which is identified by its thickened walls. **Aii** indicates the thick free wall while **Aiii** shows the position of the septal wall of the inter-ventricular septum.
(b) These are the papillary muscles which run from the internal surfaces of the ventricular walls and extend, by the continuing chordae tendineae, to the serrated edges of the atrioventricular valve cusps.
(c) This is the left auricle which receives oxygenated blood from the lungs via the pulmonary veins.
(d) This is the trabecula septomarginalis (moderator band) which runs from the septal wall near the base of the largest papillary muscle of the right ventricle to its free wall. This carries the conducting Purkinje fibres across the lumen of the right ventricular chamber. It is found only in the right ventricle.
(e) This is the mm. pectinati which is apparent on the inner surfaces of both the right and left auricles.

107. (a) This is the interior of a ventricle of the heart.
(b) **Bi** is the atrioventricular valve and **Bii** is the valve cusp.
(c) Marker **Ci** shows the semilunar valve and marker **Cii** shows the semilunar valvula.
(d) Marker **D** shows the chordae tendineae which connect the valve cusps with the papillary muscles.
(e) The thick musculature of the ventricular wall indicates that this is the left ventricle. The vessel distal to the semilunar valve has a thick elastic wall which would suggest the aorta. Thus, **Bi** is the left atrioventricular valve (mitral or bicuspid) while **Ci** is the aortic valve.

108.(a) The vessels are as follows: **Ai** — caudal, **Aii** — cranial venae cavae.
  (b) Region **Bi** is the atrium of the heart. **Bii** indicates the cusps of the atrioventricular valve.
  (c) This is the intervenous tubercle.
  (d) This is the region of the coronary sinus.
  (e) This is the area of the fossa ovalis.

Abdomen and Pelvis

109.(a) This is the fifth lumbar vertebra of a dog which is identified by the extensive transverse processes typical of the lumbar region.
  (b) Area **B** is the mamillary process.
  (c) Area **C** is the caudal articular process which forms a synovial joint with the cranial articular process of the next adjacent vertebra.
  (d) Area **D** is the caudal face of the vertebral body. This forms a cartilaginous (amphiarthrodial) joint with the next adjacent vertebral body. The intervertebral disc is found between the two faces.
  (e) This is the vertebral foramen. The spinal cord lies within its arch, enclosed in the meninges, the dura mater, the arachnoid membrane and the pia mater. The fat layer of the epidural space surrounds the dura mater.

110.(a) This is the lateral aspect of a dog sacrum which lies between the seventh lumbar and the first caudal vertebrae.
  (b) The sacrum is made up of the unification of three vertebral elements.
  (c) This is the auricular surface of the wing of the sacrum. This articulates with the wing of the ilium to form a combined synovial and cartilaginous joint. There is virtually no movement at this joint.
  (d) The prominences are: **Di** — median sacral crest, **Dii** — intermediate sacral crest.
  (e) The areas are: **Ei** — caudal face of sacral body, **Eii** — transverse process. The former articulates with the body of the first caudal vertebra but that vertebra fails to articulate its rudimentary cranial articular processes with the sacrum. The transverse processes do not articulate with the caudal vertebra.

111.(a) These are caudal vertebrae which lie in the most caudal region of the vertebral column, commencing caudal to the sacrum.
  (b) The most cranial of the group would be **Biii** as it has the most completely developed features, then in sequence **Biv**, **Bii** and **Bi** as their prominences are decreasingly obvious.
  (c) The projections are as follows: **Ci** — cranial articular process, **Cii** — mamillary process. Only the former articulates with the preceding vertebra.
  (d) This is the neural arch, which overlies the vertebral canal. At this level, the canal contains only caudal nerves enveloped in dura mater as the spinal cord has terminated at the conus medullaris in the distal lumbar region. In the later caudal vertebrae, the canal is reduced to a groove such as in vertebrae **Bi** and **Bii**.
  (e) This is the haemal arch overlying the canal which conducts the median caudal artery.

112.(a) This is the first lumbar vertebra of a dog.
  (b) These are the transverse processes of the lumbar vertebrae which give rise to the m. transversus abdominis.

(c) This is the wing of ilium.

(d) This aperture is the intervertebral foramen between the fifth and sixth lumbar vertebrae. The fifth spinal nerve emerges through it. This divides into dorsal and ventral branches — the former supplies the dorsal epaxial region, the latter runs into the lumbosacral plexus, thus supplying components to the femoral nerve of the pelvic limb.

(e) This is the vertebral canal. At this level the canal contains the spinal cord enveloped by meningeal layers of the dura mater, arachnoid membrane and pia mater. These are present at **Ei** but by the level of **Eii** the cord has terminated as the conus medullaris while the meningeal layers are forming the filum terminale. The canal contains the cauda equina.

113. (a) This is the superficial ventral abdomen of a bitch. The vulva is an obvious feature as it lies caudally under the tail.

(b) These are the teats of: **Bi** — cranial abdominal, **Bii** — caudal abdominal and **Biii** — inguinal abdominal mammary glands.

(c) This is the superficial opening of the inguinal canal through which passes the external pudendal artery and vein. The caudal superficial epigastric artery and vein of that side arise from these vessels. The latter are seen at **Cii**.

(d) This is an umbilical scar which in fetal times allowed passage of the umbilical cord from the abdominal cavity. After birth and severance of the cord, the patent aperture healed over to form the umbilical scar.

(e) This is the median raphe which is superficial to the linea alba.

114. (a) This is the m. obliquus externus abdominis which originates from costal attachments, fifth to twelfth ribs, and the thoracolumbar fascia. It inserts onto the linea alba by means of a broad aponeurosis.

(b) This is the m. rectus abdominis which originates cranially from the sternum and the first costal cartilage and rib. It inserts caudally onto the prepubic tendon.

(c) This the external inguinal opening through which the vaginal process with the external pudendal vessels can be seen emerging.

(d) This is the femoral triangle. The femoral artery and vein and the saphenous nerve, a branch of the femoral nerve, can be seen coursing through this region.

(e) This is the m. pectineus which is an adductor of the pelvic limb; it is innervated by the obturator nerve.

115. (a) This is the m. obliquus internus abdominis. The markers are as follows: **Ai** — pars costalis, which originates from the twelfth and thirteenth ribs, **Aii** — pars abdominis, which arises from the thoracolumbar fascia, **Aii** — pars inguinalis, which can be seen attaching caudally onto the inguinal ligament.

(b) This is the m. obliquus externus abdominis. This is responsible for assisting in increasing intra-abdominal pressure on contraction during functions such as expiration, defaecation, urination and parturition. It can also assist in flexion of the vertebral column.

(c) This is the m. transversus abdominis which originates from the transverse processes of the lumbar vertebrae, the tuber coxae and the eighth costal cartilage.

(d) This is the linea alba, a relatively non-vascular structure. Because of this feature and its tough fibrous nature, allowing good anchorage for sutures, it is frequently chosen as the line of incision for surgically entering the abdomen.

ANSWERS

(e) The abdominal muscles of both sides insert by aponeurotic sheets onto the midline linea alba forming the 'sheath of the rectus' around the m. rectus abdominis. The external oblique muscle sends sheets which are always external to the rectus muscle. An aponeurosis of internal oblique muscle passes internally to the rectus in the cranial third of the abdomen but then reverts to lying external to the rectus muscle. The transverse muscle has an aponeurosis which is internal to the rectus until the most caudal abdominal region and then lies external to the rectus muscle. Thus, there is no aponeurotic sheath internal to the rectus muscle in the most caudal abdomen region.

116. (a) This is the xiphoid process of the sternum.
  (b) These are the costal cartilages which run from the tenth, eleventh and twelfth ribs to form the costal arch running to join the sternum.
  (c) This is the m. transversus abdominis which is revealed by the removal of the m. obliquus externus abdominis and the m. obliquus internus abdominis.
  (d) These structures are the medial branches of the ventral divisions of the thoracic and lumbar spinal nerves.
  (e) This area has been cleared by the removal of the m. rectus abdominis to reveal the abdominal viscera seen through the aponeurosis of the m. transversus abdominis, the fascia transversalis and the parietal peritoneum.

117. (a) This is the outer surface and external lamina of the prepuce.
  (b) This is the m. preputialis, an offshoot of the m. cutaneous trunci. Its motor innervation comes from the cutaneous branches of the ventral branches of the eighth cervical and the first thoracic nerves.
  (c) This is the pars longa glandis of the penis.
  (d) This is the bulbus glandis of the penis. This receives blood from the internal pudendal artery via the dorsal artery and the deep artery of the penis. It also receives additional supply from the external pudendal artery via the preputial branch of the penile dorsal artery.
  (e) This is the scrotum of a male dog which contains the testes in life. The surgical incision would be made through skin, dartos muscle, external spermatic fascia, parietal layer of vaginal tunic, visceral layer of vaginal tunic and into the tunica albuginea of the testis.

118. (a) The region described contains the prepuce in many species.
  (b) The terminal portion of the penis would be found in this space.
  (c) The marker is pointing to the opening into a recess termed the preputial diverticulum, found in the male pig.
  (d) This space contains stale foul smelling urine and cell debris in the live animal.
  (e) Area **B** is lined with modified skin although it gives appearance of a mucous membrane.

119. (a) This is the superficial inguinal opening which is formed by a slit in the aponeurosis of the m. obliquus externus abdominis. The deep inguinal opening is formed by the m. rectus abdominis medially, the m. obliquus abdominis internus cranially and the inguinal ligament caudally.
  (b) This is the spermatic cord which contains the ductus deferens, artery of the ductus deferens, testicular artery and vein, testicular nerves and testicular lymphatics. All of this is covered by the vaginal process.

146

(c) **Ci** shows the right testis, enveloped by the parietal layer of the vaginal tunic. At **Cii**, the left testis is visualised by resection of the parietal layer to expose the testis covered only by the visceral layer of vaginal tunic.

(d) This is the m. cremaster which draws the scrotal contents closer to the abdominal wall. It is an offshoot of the m. obliquus abdominis internus.

(e) This is the ductus deferens as it courses from its origin at the tail of the epididymis to enter the pelvic urethra at the neck of the bladder.

120. (a) This is the external opening of the inguinal canal.

(b) This slit occurs in the aponeurosis of the m. obliquus externus abdominis.

(c) This is the cremaster muscle, which is composed of striated muscle. This muscle originates from the m. obliquus internus abdominis and inserts into the parietal vaginal tunic of the scrotal region.

(d) Muscle **C** overlies the spermatic cord as it emerges from the inguinal opening.

(e) This is the body of the penis.

121. (a) This is the tail or extremitas caudata of the testis.

(b) This is the head of the epididymis.

(c) This structure is the ductus deferen. **Cii** shows the lateral, **Ciii** shows the medial aspect of the testis. The ductus deferens is visible running along the caudomedial border of the testis.

(d) **Di** is the proper ligament of the testis, **Dii** is the ligament of the tail of the epididymis. Only the latter must be severed in an open castration to release the testis from the scrotal sac and the parietal layer of the vaginal tunic. In a closed castration, neither is cut as only the scrotal ligament need be severed to allow the testis to be removed within an intact vaginal tunic.

(e) This is the pampiniform plexus of testicular veins which encircle the testicular artery. The mesh of veins act as a thermoregulatory device permitting cooling of arterial blood by heat exchange before it enters the testis.

122. (a) The testis is shown in longitudinal section in **Ai** and in cross-section in **Aii**.

(b) This is the tunica albuginea which is covered on its outer surface by the visceral layer of the vaginal tunic.

(c) This region is the mediastinum testis which is a cord of connective tissue containing the straight tubules, testicular vessels and lymphatics.

(d) This is the epididymis, where storage and maturation of spermatozoa takes place.

(e) This is the ductus deferens which arises from the tail of the epididymis, **Eiii**.

123. (a) This is the testis

(b) This is the head of the epididymis which in this case is pigmented. The head is encroaching onto the free border of the testis which, accompanied by its wide girth and pigmentation, indicates that this is the testis of a ram.

(c) This is the tail of the epididymis, a well rounded structure, lying most ventrally on the testis as it hangs vertically within the dependent scrotum of the ruminant. The duct of the epididymis passes through the epididymis to its tail and then exits as the ductus deferens.

(d) This is the parietal layer of the vaginal tunic as it runs onto the surface of the testis as the visceral layer to form the ligament of the epididymal tail.

(e) This is the m. cremaster which is striated muscle. It originates from the parent m. obliquus internus abdominis.

ANSWERS

124. (a) This is a testis which has been cut in the median plane to reveal a section through the organ from its head to the tail and epididymis.
(b) The outermost layers comprise the visceral layer of the vaginal tunic, serous membrane and the inner tunica albuginea which is a fibrous coat.
(c) These layers are septa which divide the parenchyma of the testis into lobules. The parenchyma contains the seminiferous tubules, which are lined by the spermatogenic cells, and the sustentacular cells. The glandular cells (formerly the interstitial cells of Leydig) are found in the interlobular connective tissue.
(d) This is the mediastinum testis, a mass of fibrous tissue receiving the continuation of the seminiferous tubules, the straight tubules, which unite within the mediastinum to form the rete testis.
(e) The rete testis carries the spermatozoa from the mediastinum towards the head of the testis from where they leave the testis to enter the head of the epididymis via the efferent ductules.

125. (a) This is the testis. The organ has been revealed by cutting through the following structures in order: skin, tunica dartos, external spermatic fascia and tunica vaginalis parietalis.
(b) The markers are as follows: **Bi** — head, **Bii** — tail of epididymis.
(c) This is the ductus deferens which terminates in the pelvic urethra.
(d) This section would sever the following: testicular artery and vein, deferential artery and the vascular supply of the cremaster muscle.
(e) The pigmented head of the epididymis overlying the free border of the testis and the prominent tail of the epididymis suggests a ruminant. The testis is also somewhat spherical, indicating a small ruminant. The testis is suspended with its long axis hanging vertically in the scrotum. Thus, structures at **Di** and **Dii** would lie at the neck of the scrotum, situated in an inguinal position. Structures from each scrotal sac would pass on either side of the body of penis, immediately caudal to the sigmoid flexure.

126. (a) The markers are as follows: **Ai** — testis, **Aii** — free border, **Aiii** — cranial extremity, **Aiv** — caudal extremity.
(b) The markers are as follows: **Bi** — body, **Bii** — head, **Biii** — tail of epididymis.
(c) Marker **Ci** overlies the visceral layer of the vaginal tunic and the tunica albuginea of the testis. **Cii** indicates various whorls of testicular vessels in the tunica albuginea.
(d) This is the m. cremaster which is responsible for pulling the testis closer to the abdominal body wall.
(e) The testis has a long oval shape, not spherical, and the epididymis extends onto the free border of the testis at its cranial extremity. The tail of the epididymis is large and rounded, projecting well away from the caudal extremity. The whorls of vessels are characteristic of a ruminant and the angle of the long axis relative to the m. cremaster would indicate a testis which hung vertically, the caudal extremity being ventral in position. All these facts indicate a bull testis.

127. (a) This is the epididymal border of the testis.
(b) This is the ductus deferens, which conveys sperm from the tail of the epididymis to the pelvic urethra.
(c) This is the spermatic cord. The pampiniform plexus, an extensive plexus of testicular veins arranged around the artery, can be seen. This has a thermoregulatory mechanism.

(d) This is the proper ligament of the testis.

(e) The testis is long and oval while the head of the epididymis overlies the free border of the testis. These observations, together with the whorls of veins beneath the tunica albuginea, are indicative of a bull. The testis also hangs vertically from the region of the spermatic cord, again typical of a ruminant. The ductus deferens lies on the caudomedial aspect of the testis. Thus, this is the medial face of the organ.

128.(a) This is a testis. **Ai** is the epididymal border, **Aii** is the free border.

(b) The markers are as follows: **Bi** — tail, **Bii** — head of the epididymis.

(c) The testis is long and elliptical. It has straight vessels in the tunica albuginea rather than whorls and the head of the epididymis does not encroach on the free border of the testis. This suggests a porcine organ.

(d) Boar testes lie caudally in the prominent scrotal sac just ventral to the anal opening.

(e) The long axis of the testis is almost horizontal so that the tail of the epididymis, **Bi**, is directed caudally and the head, **Bii**, cranially.

129.(a) This is the testis of a boar.

(b) This is the tail of the epididymis.

(c) **Ci** is the ductus deferens which conveys spermatozoa from the tail of the epididymis to the pelvic urethra. **Cii** is the mesorchium, which connects the gonad with the parietal layer of the vaginal tunic.

(d) This is the proper ligament of the testis.

(e) This is the ligament of the tail of the epididymis.

130.(a) This is a testis. Marker **A** shows the tunica albuginea.

(b) The strands of tissue are the septa which run from the outer tunic towards the centre of the organ. The parenchyma of the lobules lying between these septa contains the seminiferous tubules which contain the spermatogonia and the sustentacular cells. The glandular cells lie in the interlobular tissue.

(c) This is the mediastinum which contains the rete testis.

(d) Marker **Di** shows the efferent ductules which leave the testis at **Dii** to join the head of the epididymis.

(e) The very distinct fibrous nature of the septa and the well defined mediastinum are indicative of a porcine testis. This is further justified by the long elliptical shape of the organ with its strong colouration and wide mesorchium.

131.(a) This is the m. obliquus abdominis externus which has muscle fibres running in a caudoventral direction.

(b) This is the m. obliquus abdominis internus which has muscle fibres running in a cranioventral direction.

(c) This is the m. transversus abdominis which has muscle fibres running in a transverse direction and has ventral divisions of thoracic and lumbar spinal nerves coursing across its surface.

(d) If the m. transversus abdominis were to be sectioned the parietal peritoneum would be encountered before entering into the peritoneal cavity within the abdomen.

(e) A pair of forceps advanced into the wound might encounter the left ovary and uterine horn which lie immediately caudal to the left kidney.

132.(a) This is a spleen.

(b) This is a liver. **Bi** is the left medial and **Bii** the left lateral lobes.

(c) This is a left kidney.

(d) This is the descending colon which lies on the left as it passes caudally through the abdominal cavity.

(e) This is the stomach with the marker overlying the fundic region.

133. (a) This is the descending duodenum.

(b) This is the pancreas.

(c) These are coils of jejunum as seen through the layers of the greater omentum.

(d) The markers are as follows: **Di** — right medial, **Dii** — right lateral lobes of the liver.

(e) This is the right kidney which is seen lying partially embedded in the caudate process of the caudate lobe.

134. (a) This is the ventral extremity of the spleen.

(b) These are coils of jejunum as seen through the layers of greater omentum.

(c) The markers are as follows: **Ci** — right medial, **Cii** — left lateral, **Ciii** — quadrate, **Civ** — left medial lobes of liver.

(d) This is the greater curvature of the stomach seen extending beyond the ventral border of the left lateral lobe of the liver.

(e) This is the falciform ligament. This fat-laden structure runs between the ventral abdominal floor at the level of the umbilicus and the liver.

135. (a) This is the greater omentum. This attaches to the greater curvature of the stomach and hilus of the spleen via its offshoot, the gastrosplenic ligament. The greater omentum has been reflected by lifting its caudal border (as it is not attached here) and pulling cranially. Nothing has been sectioned.

(b) This is the jejunum.

(c) This is the duodenum which descends from a cranial position at its origin from the pylorus to run to the caudal flexure where it starts to ascend cranially but in a more medial location.

(d) This is the urinary bladder showing the median ligament of the bladder stretching from its ventral surface to extend to the ventral abdominal wall.

(e) This is the diaphragm with the liver lying immediately caudal to it. The liver attaches to the diaphragm by a series of peritoneal reflections, the coronary and the triangular ligaments of liver.

136. (a) This is the ascending duodenum which travels from its caudal flexure to ascend cranially to become confluent with the jejunum.

(b) This is the right limb of the pancreas which lies in the fold of the mesoduodenum.

(c) The markers are as follows: **Ci** — caecum, **Cii** — ascending colon. The area gains arterial flow cranially from the cranial mesenteric artery and caudally from the caudal mesenteric artery.

(d) This is the ileum, the terminal portion of the small intestine. The venous blood drains into the portal vein and is eventually returned to the liver to subsequently flow back into the general circulation by means of the hepatic veins into the caudal vena cava.

(e) This is the great mesentery. This bears the mesenteric arteries flowing to the jejunum, mesenteric veins flowing to the portal vein and therefore the liver and mesenteric lymphatics which are draining into the mesenteric lymph nodes and then into the cisterna chyli at the level of crura of diaphragm.

137.(a) This is the parietal surface of the stomach at the greater curvature. Arterial blood flow would be from the coeliac artery by means of gastric and splenic arteries.

(b) This section has removed the caecum and ileum as this is the level of the ileocolic junction where the small and large intestine join.

(c) The markers are as follows: **Ci** — transverse, **Cii** — descending colon, both of which lie supported by the mesocolon.

(d) This is the spleen with the gastrosplenic ligament attaching to its hilus.

(e) The arterial blood flow to the organ is by the splenic artery which is derived from the coeliac artery from the aorta. The venous return is via the splenic vein to the liver by means of the portal vein.

138.(a) Marker **Ai** indicates the right kidney while **Aii** indicates the caudate process of the caudate lobe of the liver which is related to **Ai** cranially.

(b) These organs are the adrenal glands which are crossed by the phrenicoabdominal artery and vein.

(c) The markers are as follows: **Ci** — left kidney, **Cii** — ureters of each side of the abdomen. The ureters run from the hilus of the kidneys to flow into the neck of the urinary bladder.

(d) These are the testicular artery and vein of the right side of the abdomen. These course from the testis, in the scrotal sac, through the inguinal canal into the abdominal cavity and then pass cranially. The vein joins either the caudal vena cava or the renal vein while the artery arises from the dorsal aorta.

(e) This is the caudal vena cava which is returning venous blood to the heart from the hind end of the animal, excluding the intestinal tract. At this level, it would be receiving blood from **Ci**, the left kidney, via the renal vein but it would not yet have received blood from **Aii**, the liver, as the hepatic veins only join the vena cava at the level of diaphragm.

139.(a) This is the stomach.

(b) This is the caecum.

(c) This is the ascending or great colon.

(d) This is the descending or small colon.

(e) This is the small intestine, the jejunum. The species is a horse.

140.(a) Ai is the caecum of a horse. Aii shows sacculations of the muscular wall, each termed an haustra, Aiii shows a muscular band termed a taenia.

(b) **Bi** is the ascending or great colon. **Bii** is the pelvic flexure, narrowed with one taenial band, **Biii** is the left ventral colon, **Biv** is the right dorsal colon.

(c) This is the ileum which enters into the base of the caecum at a narrow opening, the ileal orifice, which is in the centre of an elevation, the papilla ilealis.

(d) This is the terminal descending or small colon which becomes the rectum. This contains faecal balls in life.

(e) **Ei** is the stomach, **Eii** is the saccus caecus.

141.(a) These are coils of ascending colon which has the appearance of a conical spiral.

(b) Marker **Bi** shows the caecum and marker **Bii** shows the longitudinal muscular band (taenia) which produces sacculations of the caecal wall.

(c) Structure **Ci** is the jejunum, **Cii** is the terminal ileum of the small intestine.

(d) This is the great mesentery which carries the following: mesenteric arteries from the cranial mesenteric artery, mesenteric veins running to the portal vein, lymphatics which run to the mesenteric lymph nodes and then the cisterna chyli, and mesenteric nerve trunks from the vagus and sympathetic trunk.

(e) The conical spiral of the ascending colon, taenial bands of the caecum and the straight pattern of the vascular trunks in the great mesentery all indicate a set of porcine viscera.

142. (a) This is the spleen.

(b) These are coils of ascending colon.

(c) The colon is in the shape of a flattened coil which would indicate a ruminant and as the spleen is oval in shape this suggests a bovine set of viscera.

(d) The organs are as follows: **Di** — reticulum, which is related to the entrance of the oesophagus at the cardia, **Dii** — rumen, which has the spleen applied to its dorsal sac, **Diii** — abomasum, which has the greater omentum attaching along its greater curvature.

(e) The abomasum is very large compared with the relative size of the rumen. This suggest that this was an animal which was not dependent on a herbivorous diet, i.e. a calf which would still be suckling and diverting the fluids directly into the abomasum.

143. (a) The markers are as follows: **Ai** — liver, **Aii** — notch for the round ligament, **Aii** — the caudate process of the caudate lobe.

(b) The markers are as follows: **Bi** — abomasum, **Bii** — lesser curvature, **Biii** — pyloric part of the organ.

(c) **Ci** is the omasum, **Cii** is a fold of serous membrane, the peritoneum. This specific region of peritoneum is called the lesser omentum which is seen passing from the omasum to the lesser curvature of the abomasum.

(d) **Di** shows coils of small intestine, the jejunum. **Dii** shows the great mesentery, carrying mesenteric arteries and veins, the mesenteric arteries are from the cranial mesenteric artery while the latter flows into the portal vein.

(e) The viscera are from a neonate ruminant, a calf. The liver has a large caudate process and still shows the patent vessel of an umbilical vein remnant running into the notch for the round ligament at **Aii**. The abomasum is relatively large compared with the forestomachs. The fat in the peritoneal layers is soft, grey and somewhat gelatinous indicating a very young calf.

144. (a) **Ai** is the right ovary which is held in position by the fold of suspensory ligament of the ovary, **Aii**.

(b) These vessels are the ovarian artery and vein. The former arises from the dorsal aorta, while the vein commonly drains into the caudal vena cava. These vessels are responsible for blood flow to and from the ovary and the more cranial end of the uterine horn of that side.

(c) The ligaturing of the ovarian artery and vein would be insufficient to avoid haemorrhage from the ovarian resection as some blood is received via the ascending supply of the uterine artery. It would therefore be necessary to ligature the latter vessel more distally.

(d) This is the left uterine horn which is supported by the mesometrium.

(e) This is the inguinal ring at the internal opening of the inguinal canal through which is passing the round ligament, an offshoot of mesometrium. The canal offers a natural opening from the abdominal cavity through the muscles of the region, mm. obliquus externus et internus abdominis and m. rectus abdominis.

145.(a) This is a dog kidney. Other kidneys which have a similar outline and shape would be from a cat or small ruminant. The cat kidney has capsular veins visible beneath the renal capsule and a small ruminant kidney is more rounded over its greater curvature. This is a difficult deciding factor. Perirenal fat in a well nourished sheep is white and crisp and goat kidneys often have a distinguishing odour.

(b) **Bi** is the cortex with medullary rays radiating out in its stroma. The high level of vascularisation gives the darker colour. **Bii** is the medulla which contains numerous tubules and is whiter in colour due to a lower level of vascularisation.

(c) This is the renal pelvis which collects urine.

(d) These are the interlobar arteries and veins which break up to form the arcuate vessels.

(e) The tubular structure is the ureter which runs from the renal pelvis at the hilus of the kidney to enter into the neck of the urinary bladder.

146.(a) These are pig kidneys. They are smooth externally, bean shaped but flattened dorsoventrally with slightly pointed poles.

(b) This is the hilus through which course the renal artery, renal vein and the ureter.

(c) **Ci** is the cortex and **Cii** is the medulla

(d) The interior of the kidney shows only partial fusion of the lobes with individual renal papillae. These papillae shed urine into the calices (calices minores) which form part of the renal pelvis.

(e) This is the ureter which runs from the renal pelvis to the dorsal surface of the urinary bladder by traversing the abdominal cavity from a dorsal position to the more ventrally placed bladder near the pelvic brim.

147.(a) This illustrates both halves of a sectioned equine kidney. The bean shape is characteristic of a horse's left kidney with the caudal pole wider than the cranial pole.

(b) The markers are as follows: **Bi** — cortex, **Bii** — medulla.

(c) This is the renal pelvis.

(d) This is one of the terminal recesses which connect from the pelvis to run towards the poles. This is unique to the equidae.

(e) The markers are as follows: **Ei** — interlobar vessels, **Eii** — arcuate vessels.

148.(a) These are kidneys.

(b) These are horse kidneys. They have a smooth exterior which is darkish red to brown. The two kidneys (from the same animal) differ in shape and size and the surrounding fat is typically yellow and soft in texture.

(c) **Ai** is the triangular or playing card heart-shaped right kidney. **Aii** is the left kidney, which is more bean shaped, with the caudal pole being wider than the cranial pole. (Memory aid 'the heart is in the right place'.)

(d) The right kidney extends from the sixteenth rib to the first lumbar vertebra. The left extends from the seventeenth rib to the second or third lumbar vertebrae. They are related dorsally to the right and left crura of the diaphragm. The right is in contact cranially with the liver.

(e) These organs are closely related to the adrenal glands and the pancreas.

149.(a) This is a dog spleen, which displays the characteristic J shape. **A** is the visceral surface.

(b) This is the elongated hilus of the spleen.

(c) The gastrosplenic ligament, a continuation from the greater omentum, is seen attaching in the region of the hilus.

(d) Branches of splenic artery and vein can be seen coursing through the gastrosplenic ligament. The former is a branch of the coeliac artery from the dorsal aorta. The latter flows into the portal vein to run to the liver.

(e) **Ei** indicates the region which would be in contact with the tubular intestinal tract. **Eii** points to the area of contact with the stomach.

150.(a) This is the diaphragmatic surface of a dog liver.

(b) The markers are as follows: **Bi** — right lateral, **Bii** — right medial, **Biii** — left medial, **Biv** — left lateral lobes.

(c) This is the caudal vena cava which receives blood from the liver via the hepatic veins.

(d) This is the dorsal border of the liver.

(e) This is a portion of the diaphragm which is attached to the liver by means of coronary and triangular ligaments.

151.(a) This is the visceral surface of the liver of a dog

(b) **Bi** is the papillary process of the caudate lobe. **Bii** is the caudate process of the caudate lobe of the liver.

(c) This is the quadrate lobe which extends to the ventral border of the liver.

(d) **Di** is the gall bladder from which the cystic duct, **Dii**, extends. The former stores the bile which passes into and out of the gall bladder via the cystic duct.

(e) This is the lesser omentum or hepatogastric ligament. It extends from the porta of the liver to the lesser curvature of the stomach.

152.(a) This is a pig liver. The distinct lobation sugests either a pig or a carnivore. The distinct surface marking, due to the high interlobular connective tissue content — so-called Morroco leather appearance, is characteristic of a pig liver.

(b) This is a visceral surface, which lies caudally in the abdominal cavity.

(c) The regions are as follows: **Ci** — left lateral, **Cii** — left medial, **Ciii** — quadrate, **Civ** — right medial, **Cv** — right lateral lobe.

(d) This is the gall bladder which stores bile before it flows into the duodenum. Bile flows into and from the gall bladder via the cystic duct which then connects with the common bile duct allowing the egress of bile into the small intestine.

(e) This is the porta of the liver into which enters the portal vein and hepatic artery. The common bile duct and lymphatic vessels draining the liver exit this region.

153.(a) This is the caudate process of the caudate lobe of a ruminant liver. The liver is relatively non lobated and lacks interlobar notches indicating a ruminant. The caudate process is relatively small and does not protrude far beyond liver edge, suggestive of a sheep.

(b) This is the diaphragmatic surface of the liver which is directed cranially in the live animal.

(c) The marker is indicating the sectioned diaphragm and is overlying the tendinous centre of that muscle.

(d) This is the dorsal border of the liver where the oesophagus runs over the edge of the organ creating the oesophageal impression.

(e) This is the notch for the round ligament, which lies to the right of the midline in the live animal.

154.(a) This is a ruminant liver. The liver is undivided and lacks interlobar notches except for the notch for the round ligament.

(b) **Bi** is the sectioned portal vein at the region of the porta of the liver. **Bii** is the hepatogastric ligament, part of lesser omentum. Both are found on the visceral surface of the liver.

(c) This is the region from where the gall bladder has been removed. This lies on the right border of the organ, thus on the right side of the animal.

(d) **Di** is the caudate process, **Dii** is the papillary process of the caudate lobe of the liver. The relatively large caudate process protruding well beyond the dorsal edge would indicate a bovine liver.

(e) This is the vena cava revealing its interior where the perforations of the hepatic veins into its lumen are visible. This would be situated on the dorsal border of the liver.

155.(a) This is ruminant liver which lacks lobation and has no obvious interlobar notches.

(b) This is the diaphragmatic surface. Marker **B** lies on the left margin of the organ and does, in fact, indicate the region where the oesophagus passes over the liver.

(c) This is the caudate process of the caudate lobe of the liver. This is protruding considerably beyond the dorsal edge, which suggests a bovine liver.

(d) This is the notch for the round ligament. This contains the vestigial ligament in the adult and it may only be a small remnant but in the calf it may contain the degenerating umbilical vein.

(e) This is the falciform ligament coursing over the diaphragmatic surface of the liver.

156.(a) This is a sheep rumen. This has a characteristic papillated lining indicating the forestomach of a ruminant. The heavy staining and high degree of papillation would indicate an adult animal which has been existing on a herbivorous diet. The overall size is relatively small indicating a small adult ruminant, possibly a sheep. A calf would have a relatively small rumen but would be less stained and not as heavily papillated if it was still suckling.

(b) **Bi** has little papillation and appears smooth compared with **Bii**. This smooth lining is associated with the dorsal roof of the rumen as a gas bubble exists here in life with a resultant loss in papillation. One can therefore deduce that an incision has been made into the dorsal sac of the rumen allowing observation down into the ventral sac, **Biii**, which is heavily stained and papillated.

(c) These are the left and right longitudinal pillars of the rumen, which demarcate the dorsal from the ventral sac. The pillars represent foldlike duplication of the internal smooth muscle of the stomach wall and, lacking in papillae, they have a smooth, light coloured appearance.

(d) The innervation is derived from the vagus nerves which arrive in the region of the cardia after passing through the hiatus oesophageus along with the oesophagus. The sympathetic nerves which arrive through the periarterial plexuses have a minor role.

(e) The major blood supply is from the coeliac artery from the aorta. The drainage is by ruminal veins into the splenic vein, a major tributary of the portal vein running to liver.

157.(a) This is the omasum of an adult ruminant, most possibly a cow.

(b) The chamber of the omasum is the third of the three forestomachs and the third of the four stomach chambers of the ruminant.

(c) This is the omasal groove, which forms the basis of the omasal canal which represents the direct route from the reticulum to the abomasum.

(d) These structures are the omasal laminae. These are covered by a mucous membrane studded with short stubby papillae.

(e) These spaces are the interlaminar recesses which contain further laminae of varying heights which all form a series of laminae of four differing relative heights. There would be ingesta trapped in the recesses in life.

158.(a) The incision has been made into the forestomachs of an adult ruminant, most possibly a cow.

(b) **Bi** indicates the typical honeycomb-like cells of the lining of the reticulum. **Bii** indicates the pile-like appearance of the tongue-shaped papillae covering the interior of the rumen.

(c) This is the cardia which has a whiter appearance than the surrounding area due to a relative lack of papillation. It is the point of entrance for swallowed ingesta and also the point of exit for regurgitated material returning to the oral cavity during rumination in adult.

(d) This is the reticular groove, which connects the cardia with the reticulo-omasal opening. It is the first part of the gastric groove which allows fluid to be diverted from the cardia straight through to the abomasum in the suckling calf.

(e) These are thin curved papillae found in the groove, the papillae unguliformes.

159.(a) The markers are as follows: **Ai** — dorsal sac, **Aii** — caudoventral blind sac, **Aiii** — ventral sac of the rumen.

(b) The markers are as follows: **Bi** — ventral coronary groove, **Bii** — right longitudinal groove.

(c) The markers are as follows: **Ci** — fundus, **Cii** — greater curvature, **Ciii** — pyloric part of abomasum.

(d) This is the reticulum which lies in a cranial position; it is in apposition with the liver and the diaphragm and thus indirectly with the pericardium.

(e) This is the omasum which interconnects directly with **C**, the abomasum, and **D**, the reticulum.

160.(a) This is the reticulum which lies in apposition cranially with the liver and the diaphragm.

(b) This is the omasum which lies under the eighth to the tenth ribs, mid-ventrally in the abdominal cavity and to the right of the midline.

(c) The markers are: **Ci** — dorsal sac, **Cii** — ventral sac, **Ciii** — caudodorsal blind sac, **Civ** — caudoventral blind sac of the rumen. This is the left side of the organ.

(d) This furrow is the left dorsal coronary groove which contains ruminal arteries, veins and nerves. The arteries arise from the coeliac artery, the nerves arise from the vagus nerve (X). The veins eventually flow into the portal vein.

(e) This is the oesophagus which has a striated muscular wall. This region of the organ would receive blood flow from either the coeliac artery or the broncho-oesophageal artery.

161.(a) This is the ventral surface of the ventral sac of the rumen.

(b) This is the reticulum.

(c) The markers are as follows: **Ci** — body, **Cii** — pyloric part of the abomasum.

(d) This is the liver.

(e) **Ei** is the superficial leaf of the greater omentum, overlying the coils of the small intestine, i.e. the jejunum. The latter is lying in the supraomental recess.

162.(a) This is the cardia of a dog stomach which lies in the cranial abdomen to the left of the midline where the oesophagus joins it as it passes through the diaphragm. The oesophagus has been sectioned here to allow the removal of the stomach from the abdominal cavity.

(b) This is the fundus of a dog stomach. When empty, it usually lies to the left of the midline in the cranial abdominal region in a dorsal position. After feeding, this is the stomach region which expands and may extend ventrally and caudally depending on the volume of food consumed.

(c) This is the pylorus of the stomach. This is usually found to the right of the midline in the cranial abdominal region.

(d) This is the descending duodenum which lies dorsolaterally, to the right of the midline in the abdominal cavity.

(e) These are the right and left lobes of the pancreas which acts as both an endocrine (insulin) and exocrine gland. The exocrine secretion travels via two ducts to open into the duodenum immediately distal to the pylorus. The right lobe lies adjacent to the descending duodenum in the mesoduodenum.

163.(a) This is a dog stomach which has been opened along its greater curvature. Marker **A** shows the cardia with cardiac glands.

(b) This is the fundus, which contains the gastric glands proper.

(c) This is the pyloric antrum and canal, which is lined with pyloric glands.

(d) This is the duodenum which is lined with a mucous coat. This has a velvety appearance on its free surface due to the presence of innumerable intestinal villi.

(e) The probe is in a major duodenal papilla onto which open the bile and pancreatic ducts. **Eii** is a minor duodenal papilla onto which opens the accessory pancreatic duct.

164.(a) This is a simple stomach.

(b) This is a sectioned oesophagus which enters the stomach at the cardia.

(c) This is the duodenum, which exits from the stomach at the pylorus.

(d) **Di** is the greater curvature, **Dii** is the lesser curvature, **Diii** is the blind sac or saccus caecus.

(e) This organ is from a horse. The saccus caecus, the extremely short lesser curvature and the bright yellow fat are all characteristic of the equine stomach.

165.(a) This is the interior of a simple stomach with a composite lining.

(b) **Bi** is the cardia, **Bii** is the extensive proventricular part of the gastric mucosa.

(c) This is the margo plicatus which separates the proventricular part from the glandular part of the gastric mucosa. This feature, together with the extensive whitish non-glandular proventricular part in a simple stomach with a composite lining are all indicative of an equine stomach.

(d) **Di** is the pyloric part of the stomach, **Dii** is the pyloric sphincter which is situated at the point of exit from the stomach.

(e) **Ei** is the duodenum, **Eii** is the major duodenal papilla where the bile and pancreatic ducts enter.

166.(a) This is the parietal surface of the spleen.

(b) **Bi** is the simple stomach, **Bii** is an area where the stomach is overlaid by a fold of peritoneum, the gastrosplenic ligament.

(c) This region is the gastric diverticulum.

ANSWERS

(d) The distinct pouch-like diverticulum near the cardiac region of a simple stomach and the long, narrow, strap-like spleen are characteristic of a pig.
(e) **Ei** is the duodenum, **Eii** is the pancreas.

167. (a) This is a simple stomach with a composite lining.
(b) This is the cardia where the oesophagus opens into the stomach.
(c) This is the proventricular part of the gastric mucosa, which is aglandular in nature.
(d) This is the gastric diverticulum, which is demarcated from the fundic region by a distinct muscular fold. Its appearance in a stomach with a composite lining including an aglandular region immediately around the cardia suggest a porcine stomach.
(e) **Ei** is the region of the cardiac glands, **Eii** is the fundus with the region of the proper gastric glands, **Eiii** is the pyloric part with the pyloric gland region. **Eiv** is the torus pyloricus, an elevation of adipose and muscle tissue, protruding into the lumen of the pyloric canal.

168. (a) This is the ileum, which is recognised by a narrower diameter and velvety mucous lining with microvilli.
(b) This is the ascending colon, which is recognised by the greater diameter and whiter appearance of the non-villous mucous membrane.
(c) This is the caecum, which is coiled in appearance indicating a dog. Larger animal species have much enlarged caeca while cats have a simple uncoiled organ.
(d) This is the caecocolic orifice which connects the caecum with the proximal portion of the colon.
(e) The marker is indicating the fold of tissue which formed the sphincter at the ileocolic orifice.

169. (a) This is a cat kidney with capsular veins apparent on the surface which appear as vascular whorls.
(b) This is a cat spleen with the parietal surface exposed.
(c) This is a cat liver with the visceral surface exposed.
(d) This structure is the gall bladder. This is surrounded by the quadrate lobe of the liver on the left and the medial lobe on the right.
(e) This is the porta which allows passage of the portal vein and hepatic artery into the liver and the common bile duct together with the lymphatic vessels from the liver.

170. (a) This is the spleen.
(b) The parietal face of the spleen is shown here.
(c) This is an equine organ. It is triangular with a broad dorsal end and a pointed ventral extremity, it is also bluish in colour.
(d) This is closely associated with the stomach in life.
(e) This organ lies against the left abdominal wall deep to the ribs. The ventral end reaches to the ninth to eleventh intercostal spaces. The dorsal end extends caudally to the transverse process of the first lumbar vertebra.

171. (a) This is the visceral surface of a spleen.
(b) **Bi** would lie ventrally, **Bii** would be directed dorsally.
(c) This is the characteristic elongated hilus of an equine spleen with the gastrosplenic ligament attached to it.
(d) This is the splenic artery, a branch of the coeliac artery from the aorta.
(e) **Ei** is an area of attachment for the renosplenic ligament which runs to the left kidney. **Eii** is the origin of the phrenicosplenic ligament which attaches to the diaphragm.

158

172.(a) This is a cross-sectioned kidney showing the colour difference between the exterior band of the cortex and the interior layer of the medulla.

(b) This is the caudate process of the caudate lobe of the liver with the right kidney recessed into its substance. The marker is on the right because the right kidney lies in close association with the liver while the left is more caudal in position and therefore not so closely related to the liver.

(c) **Ci** is the dorsal extremity of the spleen and **Cii** is the caudal extremity of the spleen.

(d) This is the descending limb of the duodenum which lies on the extreme right of the abdominal cavity.

(e) This is a portion of the greater omentum which overlies the m. transversus abdominis and the more externally placed m. rectus abdominis.

173.(a) This is the rectum which has been imaged as it runs caudally.

(b) This is the transverse colon imaged as it lies cranial to the cranial mesenteric artery.

(c) This is the caecum which lies adjacent to the ascending colon as it runs cranially to join the transverse colon.

(d) The marker lies on the left-hand side of the abdomen. The descending colon, which lies immediately cranial to the marker, is found on this side of the abdomen.

(e) This is the anus which overlies the pelvic symphysis, consisting of the midline union of the pubes and ischii.

174.(a) **Ai** is the uterine horn of a pregnant bitch. **Aii** and **Aiii** are placed on the loci of the conceptuses where there is an enlargement of the diameter of the horn.

(b) This is the ovary which has several surface corpora lutea indicating the possibility of pregnancy. This observation, coupled with the enlarged uterine horn, both support this theory.

(c) **Ci** is the mesometrium (broad ligament). **Cii** is the round ligament. The former attaches to the dorsolateral abdominal wall and the tubular uterine tract. The latter, an offshoot of the mesometrium, runs from the region of uterine tube to the vaginal ring at the inguinal canal, through which it traverses.

(d) This is the vagina which lies at the pubic brim at the pelvic inlet.

(e) These are the right uterine artery and vein. When resecting the uterus, it is necessary not only to ligate the uterine vessels but also the ovarian vessels, which lie cranially in the mesovarium on each side.

175.(a) **Aii** is the cervix which marks the junction between the uterine body, **Ai**, and the vagina, **Aiii**.

(b) **Bi** is the vestibule. The areas of the vestibular bulbs are indicated by the markers **Bii**.

(c) This is the external urethral orifice through which passes urine on its journey from the urinary bladder to the vestibule and thus the exterior via the vulva.

(d) **Di** is the clitoris, **Dii** is the fossa clitoridis.

(e) **Ei** is the endometrial lining of the uterine horn. The colour variations are because this is the uterus of a pregnant bitch and **Eii** overlays a region where the zonary placenta has been attached.

176.(a) These organs belong to the female urogenital system.

(b) The markers are as follows: **Bi** — uterine horn, **Bii** — body of uterus, **Biii** — region of cervix.

(c) These are the left and right ovaries. Their appearance differs as **Ci** is still covered by the mesovarium while in **Cii** the ovarian bursa has been rolled back to expose the ovary.

(d) This is the uterine tube, the proximal end of which lies adjacent to the ovary, being termed the infundibulum. The distal end merges into the uterine horn.

(e) The long convoluted uterine horn, the long cervical region and the ovary with multiple structures on its surface all indicate that this is the tract of a sow. The ovary is obviously active and the uterine horn has a significant diameter with a reasonably extensive mesometrium. This would indicate a mature sow that is cycling and has had previous litters of piglets.

177. (a) **Ai** is the uterine body, **Aii** is the uterine horn, which displays the presence of caruncles through the wall, **Aiii** is the uterine tube.

(b) **Bi** is the ovary, **Bii** is the corpus luteum which contains luteal tissue essential for the establishment and perpetuation of pregnancy.

(c) This is the ovarian artery which comes directly off the aorta. It runs in the mesovarium along with the proper ligament of the ovary.

(d) This is the urinary bladder which collects urine from the kidneys via the ureters, voids it to the exterior via the urethra into the region of the floor of the vestibule and eventually through the vulva.

(e) The short uterine body compared with the length of the uterine horns and the simple oval-shaped ovary would indicate the female reproductive tract of a ruminant. The presence of caruncles and a corpus luteum in each ovary would suggest that this was an animal pregnant with twins. The dimension of the two gravid uterine horns and the occurrence of twins would indicate a sheep.

178. (a) This is the female urogenital system.

(b) The markers are as follows: **Bi** — uterine horn, **Bii** — uterine body, **Biii** — cervix.

(c) These are caruncles on the uterine endometrium. In a pregnant animal they would be related to the cotyledons of the placental layers.

(d) **Di** is the fold of the mesometrium (broad ligament), **Dii** is the round ligament of the uterus.

(e) These are the ovaries, which are small and oval in shape. The uterine horns are relatively long compared with the body and there is pigmentation in the interior of the horns. This suggests a sheep uterus. The ovary is relatively inactive but shows evidence of previous activity and the presence of formed caruncles indicates that the tract was from an adult non-pregnant ewe.

179. (a) This is the uterus. Marker **A** is overlying the placental layer of the chorioallantois.

(b) This is the umbilical cord, which contains the umbilical artery, the umbilical veins and the urachus.

(c) These are the cotyledons which, in life, are related to the maternal caruncles.

(d) **Di** is the genital tubercle which is placed in a perineal position indicating that the fetus, **Dii**, would be a female in life.

(e) This is the allantoic sac which contains excreted fetal urine, it is connected to the foetus by the urachus.

180. (a) This is the ovary.

(b) The finger is inserted into the ovulation fossa of the ovary.

(c) The fossa represents the confined space at which all ovulations occur in this ovary. This indicates an equine organ.

(d) This is the infundibulum which bears the abdominal opening of the uterine tube.

(e) This fold of tissue is part of the mesovarium.

181.(a) These are ovaries.

(b) These protrusions are corpora lutea.

(c) The corpora lutea represent temporary endocrine glands which produce progesterone post-ovulation and continue to do so if pregnancy ensues. They are formed on the sites of the ovulated follicles.

(d) The mesovarium has been sectioned to expose the ovary which is therefore opening into the ovarian bursa.

(e) The ovary bears multiple corpora lutea which suggests a species which has multiple offspring. To reveal the surface of the ovary, it was necessary to section the mesovarium to enter the ovarian bursa. In most species the ovary can be rolled out of the ovarian bursa without having to cut into it. The exception is in the bitch. This evidence indicates a canine ovary.

182.(a) This is the pelvic symphysis, the midline union of the pubic bones and ischii of each side.

(b) This is the urinary bladder. It is maintained in this position in the caudal abdomen and at the pelvic inlet by two lateral ligaments and an ventral ligament. These are folds of peritoneum.

(c) This is the prostate which lies dorsal to and encompasses the urethra. The organ lying dorsal to it is the rectum which can be restricted within the confines of the pelvic inlet by an enlarged prostate. This causes straining and difficulty in defaecation.

(d) This is the bulbus glandis, a region of the penis which is highly vascularised, and contains much cavernous tissue.

(e) This is the os penis which has a ventral groove which contains the penile urethra. Obstruction of the urethra usually occurs in the dog at the level immediately proximal to the os penis because at this point the tubular passageway is suddenly confined to a rigid narrow channel.

183.(a) This is a male urogenital system.

(b) This is the urinary bladder which, depending on its degree of fullness, lies at the pelvic brim or in the caudal abdomen.

(c) This is the vesicular gland.

(d) This is the bulbourethral gland.

(e) This is the body of the penis. This has a distinct spiral shape which, together with the large paired elongated bulbourethral glands and a large vesicular gland, indicates a pig. The size and advanced degree of development of these glands also indicates that this was an entire male. In the castrate, the secondary sex glands are relatively undeveloped.

184.(a) This is the male urogenital system.

(b) This is a penis.

(c) This is the glans penis.

(d) This is the external urethral orifice.

(e) The distinct spiral formed by the penis and the urethral opening eccentrically placed on the small glans indicates a porcine penis.

ANSWERS

185 (a) This is a cross-sectional face of a penis.
  (b) This is the tunica albuginea of the penis
  (c) This is the corpus cavernosum.
  (d) This is the corpus spongiosum.
  (e) This is the penile urethra through which passes urine and ejaculate at coitus. The high fibrous nature of the septa running in the penile structure would indicate a fibroelastic-type penis, this group includes the ruminant and pig.

186. (a) This is the male urogenital system.
  (b) This is the pelvic urethra which is covered by the urethralis muscle.
  (c) This is the glans of penis. The seeker is inserted into the external urethral orifice, and thus into the penile urethra.
  (d) The markers are lying at the proximal and distal extents of the sigmoid flexure of the penis.
  (e) These are two strands of the m. retractor penis. The penis is a fibroelastic type with a sigmoid flexure. There is no evidence of a secondary sex organ overhanging the pelvic urethra, as would be seen in the boar. The glans is simple in shape with no prolongation of the urethral process such as found in the small ruminant. The retractor penis muscle inserts distal to the sigmoid flexure. All these observations indicate the penis of a bull.

187. (a) **Ai** is the urinary bladder which is supported on each side by the lateral ligaments of the bladder **Aii**. The round ligaments of the bladder, **Aiii**, which are formed from the umbilical arteries, run on the cranial edge of the lateral ligaments.
  (b) These are vesicular glands which produce seminal fluid. This fluid travels via the left and right ducts to open into the pelvic urethra at the colliculus seminalis.
  (c) The incision would reveal the cut urethralis muscle and prostate gland surrounding the lumen of the pelvic urethra.
  (d) The incision would cut into the bulbourethral glands which lie deep to the m. bulbospongiosus, marked **D**.
  (e) These are the ductus deferens at level of the expanded ampulla. The firm compact irregularly elongated vesicular gland and the compact prostate gland with the concealed bulbourethral glands indicates the organs of a bull.

188. (a) These are the ischiatic tuberosities, which form part of the ischium.
  (b) This is the m. coccygeus. This arises from the ischiatic spine and inserts onto the transverse processes of the second to fifth caudal vertebrae.
  (c) This the the m. levator ani. This arises from the medial edge of the body of the ilium, from the inner surface of the ramus of the pubis and the pelvic symphysis. It inserts onto the haemal process of the seventh caudal vertebra.
  (d) Collectively, these muscles are referred to as the pelvic diaphragm. Acting together they produce compression of the rectum during defaecation.
  (e) This is sacrotuberous ligament which connects the sacrum and the ischiatic tuberosity of the ischium.

189. (a) This is the m. bulbospongiosus which overlies the bulb of the penis.
  (b) This is the m. ischiocavernosus of each side which originate, left and right, from the ischial tuberosity and insert onto the corpus cavernosum of the penis.
  (c) This is the m. retractor penis. The motor nerve supply is via the perineal branches of the pudendal nerve.

(d) This is the testis which is covered by the external spermatic fascia adhering to the parietal vaginal tunic. The scrotal wall has been cut.

(e) This is the spermatic cord. This contains the ductus deferens, the artery of the ductus deferens, the testicular artery and vein, the testicular nerves and lymphatics.

190. (a) This is the anus which is controlled by an external muscular sphincter of striated muscle and an internal anal sphincter of smooth muscle. Both muscles encircle the anal opening.

(b) These are openings of the ducts of the anal sacs. These sacs contain tubular glands, glands of the anal sacs, which discharge into the anal sacs themselves.

(c) The anal sacs lie laterally, to either side of the anal opening in a position between the external and internal anal sphincter muscles.

(d) These are the regions of the openings of the circumanal glands. In the entire male dog these may become enlarged with age and can be related to the presence of adenomas in this region.

(e) The nerve supply to this surface region is by the perineal nerves, which are branches of the pudendal nerve. The external anal sphincter receives voluntary innervation via the pudendal nerve while the internal sphincter receives parasympathetic input from the pelvic plexus and sympathetic input via the hypogastric nerve. Arterial supply is by means of the perineal arteries which are branches of the internal pudendal artery but there may be additional supply via caudal gluteal arteries.

191. (a) This is the liver.

(b) This is the kidney.

(c) This is the descending colon as it courses caudally to become the rectum.

(d) This is ingesta lying in the stomach of the dog.

(e) This is gas which is contained within coils of the small intestine, the jejunum.

Pelvic Limb

192. (a) This is the crus.

(b) This region is the pes.

(c) This prominence is the calcaneal tuberosity, which is part of the calcaneus.

(d) This elevation of skin is created by the underlying lateral saphenous vein. This forms a convenient position for venepuncture

(e) This is the ischiatic tuberosity which is part of the ischium.

193. (a) This is the greater trochanter of the femur. The gluteal muscle mass would attach here in life.

(b) The m. biceps femoris lies immediately beneath the skin surface. Its motor nerve supply is from the sciatic nerve.

(c) This is the common calcanean tendon. This is composed of tendinous input from the m. gastrocnemius, the m. flexor digitorum superficialis, the m. biceps femoris, the m. semitendinosus and the m. gracilis.

(d) **Di** overlies the lateral malleolus of the fibula. **Dii** overlies the medial malleolus of the tibia. They are therefore different bones.

(e) This is the metatarsal pad which overlies regions of the metatarsophalangeal joints of the digits. The cutaneous sensation is derived from the tibial nerve.

ANSWERS

194.(a) This is the wing of the ilium.

(b) This is the iliopubic eminence of the pubis at the region where this bone fuses with the ilium.

(c) This is the ischiatic tuberosity which is part of the ischium.

(d) The markers are as follows: **Di** — ischiatic spine, **Dii** — greater ischiatic notch, **Diii** — lesser ischiatic notch.

(e) The markers are as follows: **Ei** — symphysis pubis, **Eii** — symphysis ischii. The symphyses are fused indicating a mature dog of at least more than two years of age.

195.(a) This is the os coxae of a cat which is made up of the ilium, pubis and ischium. Strictly speaking, there is a fourth bone, the acetabular bone, which is found in the region of the acetabulum and fuses here with the other three bones. The cat has a narrow pelvis with a convex iliac crest cranially but a narrower wing of the ilium than the dog.

(b) **Bi** is the acetabular incisura which appears as a deficiency in the acetabular rim, **Bii** and **Biii**. In life, there is a transverse ligament bridging over the incisura.

(c) The markers are as follows: **Ci** — ventral pubic tubercle, **Cii** — pectin of the pubic bone, **Ciii** — iliopubic eminence. All of these are parts of the pubis and give attachment to the prepubic tendon which is a point of origin for the m. rectus abdominis and the m. pectineus.

(d) This is the region of merger of the wing with the body of the ilium. The mm. gluteus medius et profundus originates at this point.

(e) This is the site of origin of the m. rectus femoris, the long head of the m. quadriceps femoris. This head acts as a protractor of pelvic limbs, a flexor of the hip and an extensor of the stifle joint.

196.(a) **Ai** is the acetabular fossa, **Aii** is the lunate surface of the acetabulum. The latter is smooth because it is the articular surface while the fossa does not contribute to the articular area proper.

(b) **Ai** is associated with the head of the femur in the articulation of the hip joint. **Aii** receives the attachment of the ligament of the head of the femur (teres or round ligament).

(c) The bony eminences are as follows: **Ci** — cranial dorsal iliac crest, **Cii** — caudal dorsal iliac crest; both are parts of the wing of the ilium.

(d) This is the auricular surface of the sacroiliac joint. This surface, which is part of the wing of the ilium, articulates with the wing of the sacrum to form a joint which has very little movement.

(e) This is the obturator foramen. In life, it is covered over internally by the m. obturator internus and externally by the m. obturator externus.

197.(a) This is a dog femur. **Ai** is the cranial aspect, **Aii** is the caudal aspect.

(b) **Bi** is the head of the femur, **Bii** is the depression of the fovea capitis, **Biii** is the neck of the femur. **Bi** is the articular surface (it is covered by articular cartilage) of the femoral component of the hip joint meeting the lunate surface of the acetabulum. **Bii** gives attachment to the ligament of the head of the femur (teres or round ligament). **Biii** joins the head to the body of the femur and receives the distal attachment of the joint capsule of the hip joint.

(c) **Ci** is the greater trochanter, **Cii** is the lesser trochanter. The former lies laterally, the latter medially and the trochanteric fossa lies between them. They are demarcated distally by the intertrochanteric crest running between the two trochanters on the caudal aspect of the femur.

(d) This is the tochlea which receives the articular face of the patella. This sesamoid bone can be seen lying to the left of the distal extremity of the femur.

(e) These are the lateral and medial femoral condyles. They are covered by articular cartilage and are closely associated with the lateral and medial menisci as these fibrocartilaginous discs lie attached to the tibial condyles.

198.(a) The attachments are as follows: **Ai** — m. gluteus medius, **Aii** — m. gluteus profundus, **Aiii** — m. gluteus superficialis. These muscles act as extensors of the hip joint and abductors of the pelvic limb. Their motor nerve supply is the cranial and caudal gluteal nerves.

(b) The attachments are as follows: **Bi** — mm. vastus lateralis and intermedius, **Bii** — m. vastus medialis. These muscles act as extensors of the stifle joint. The motor nerve supply is the femoral nerve.

(c) **Ci** is the attachment of the m. iliacus and the m. psoas major, collectively known as the m. iliopsoas. These act as protractors of the pelvic limb and flexors of the hip. The motor nerve supply is the ventral branches of the lumbar nerves.

(d) The attachments are as follows: **Di** — lateral head of the m. gastrocnemius, **Dii** — medial head of the m. gastrocnemius, **Diii** — m. flexor digitorum superficialis. The former two muscles act as extensors of the hock or tarsal joint and the latter acts as a flexor of the digits. Their motor nerve supply is the tibial nerve.

(e) The muscles are the mm adductor magnus and brevis. These act as one muscle to produce adduction of the pelvic limb. Their motor nerve supply is the obturator nerve.

199.(a) This is a femur.

(b) This is the trochanter major.

(c) This region is the trochlear groove.

(d) This is the lateral epicondyle.

(e) This is a bovine femur. The trochanter major is extremely high and extends dorsal to the level of the femoral head. The trochlear groove has a large raised medial lip but there is no tuberosity on it proximally, as would be seen in a horse. There is no evidence of a trochanter tertius which, together with the size, would suggest a bovine origin. The trochanter major lies laterally while the trochlear groove is on cranial aspect. Therefore, this bone is from the left pelvic limb.

200.(a) This is the ilium. **Ai** marks the wing of the ilium where the auricular surface on the sacropelvic surface is articulating with the wing of the sacrum. **Aii** indicates the body of the ilium and **Aiii** shows the greater ischiatic notch.

(b) This is the ischium. **Bi** shows the ischiatic spine, **Bii** shows the lesser ischiatic notch, **Biii** shows the ischiatic tuberosity.

(c) This is the pubis. **Ci** is the iliopectineal eminence, **Cii** is the body of the pubis.

(d) This is the obturator foramen which is bounded by the pubis and the ischium.

(e) This is the femur. **Ei** marks the head of the femur located within the acetabulum. **Eii** shows the body of the femur. This is from a male dog as the os penis is evident lying between the femoral bodies at the level of marker **Eii**. The rounded contour of the scrotum can also be imaged at a most caudal position, ventral and caudal to marker **Biii**.

ANSWERS

201. (a) This is the greater trochanter of the femur.
  (b) This is the lesser trochanter of the femur.
  (c) This is the head of the femur which forms part of the hip joint. The limb is positioned in full retraction so that the joint is in extension.
  (d) This is the acetabulum which forms the articular facet of the os coxae. This region does not have a complete bony rim because there is a notch or incisura on the ventro-medial edge. This is bridged over in life by the transverse ligament but on a radiograph there is an apparent deficiency in the bone of that area.
  (e) The line is from the dorsal iliac crests which run on the dorsal border of the ilium.

202. (a) This is the m. biceps femoris which arises from the ventrocaudal end of the sacrotuberous ligament and the ischiatic tuberosity. It inserts onto the patella and through the patellar ligament to the tibial tuberosity and the cranial border of the tibia and the tuber calcanei through the common calcanean tendon. Its actions vary according to the position of the limb. It is an extensor of the hip, stifle and tarsal joint but it can also act as a flexor of the stifle. The muscle innervation is from the ischiatic (sciatic) nerve.
  (b) This is the m. tensor fasciae latae. This arises from the ventral iliac crest and inserts into the fascia lata. It acts as a flexor of the hip and extensor of the stifle. Its innervation is from the cranial gluteal nerve.
  (c) This is the m. sartorius which originates from the region cranial to the ventral iliac crest and inserts onto the cranial border of the tibia. Thus, it is a hip flexor and a protractor of the pelvic limb in addition to being a limited adductor of the thigh. The motor nerve supply is from the femoral nerve.
  (d) **Di** is the m. gluteus medialis which arises from the lateral aspect of the wing of the ilium and the dorsal crest. It inserts onto the trochanter major of the femur. It is innervated from the cranial gluteal nerve. **Dii** is the m. gluteus superficialis which arises from the gluteal fascia, the sacrum, the first caudal vertebra and the proximal end of the sacrotuberous ligament. It inserts distal to the trochanter major on the rudimentary trochanter tertius. Its innervation is the caudal gluteal nerve. Both muscles are extensors of the hip joint.
  (e) This is the point of merger of the fascia lata with the cranial border of the m. biceps femoris. An incision would reveal the m. vastus lateralis which is attached to the body of femur at this point. This is the incision used for a surgical approach to a mid-shaft femoral fracture.

203. (a) **Ai** is the m. flexor digitorum superficialis. **Aii** is the m. gastrocnemius. Both muscles arise from the caudal aspect of the distal femur but the former inserts distally on the distal phalanges while latter inserts more proximally on the calcanean tuberosity. **Ai** is both an extensor of the tarsus and a flexor of digits, but **Aii** is only an extensor of tarsus.
  (b) This is the m. tibialis cranialis which is a flexor of the tarsus. This arises from the proximal tibia and inserts onto the second and third metatarsal bones.
  (c) This is the m. extensor digitorum longus which is an extensor of the digits and a flexor of the tarsus. This muscle arises from the lateral epicondyle of the femur. The tendon of origin runs in the extensor fossa of the femur. The muscle inserts onto the distal phalanges.
  (d) This is the m. flexor hallucis longus (lateral head of the m. flexor digitorum profundus). This is a flexor of the digits and an extensor of the tarsus.

(e) **Ei** is the common peroneal (fibular) nerve, **Eii** is the tibial nerve. If the peroneal nerve was sectioned muscles **B** and **C** would be affected but **Ai**, **Aii** and **D** would still contract as they receive motor supply from the tibial nerve. Section of the peroneal nerve would result in loss of cutaneous sensation over the craniolateral region of the stifle and crus and over the dorsolateral area of the tarsus and pes.

204. (a) This is the m. semitendinosus which arises from the ischiatic tuberosity and inserts onto the medial surface of the tibia. It also contributes to the common calcanean tendon, thus inserting onto the tuber calcanei. This muscle produces extension of the hip and tarsal joint, flexion of the stifle and retraction of the pelvic limb. Its motor nerve supply is from the ischiatic (sciatic) nerve.

(b) This is the m. semimembranosus which arises from the ischiatic tuberosity and inserts onto the distal femur and the proximal tibia. It extends the hip, flexes the stifle and retracts the pelvic limb. The motor nerve supply is by the ischiatic (sciatic) nerve.

(c) This is the m. adductor. It arises from the pelvic symphysis and ischiatic arch and inserts extensively onto the caudal aspect of the femur. It is a limb adductor and its innervation is from the obturator nerve.

(d) **Di** is the m. rectus femoris and **Dii** is the m. vastus lateralis. The former arises from the body of the ilium and the latter from the femur. Both insert by a common tendon onto the patella and thus the tibial tuberosity, producing extension of the stifle joint. **Di** also acts as a flexor of the hip joint. The motor nerve is the femoral nerve.

(e) **Ei** is the ischiatic (sciatic) nerve. This bifurcates distally to give the common peroneal (fibular) nerve, **Eii** and the tibial nerve, **Eiii**.

205. (a) This is the m. pectineus which originates from the prepubic tendon and inserts onto the distal medial surface of the femur. It is an adductor of the limb. The innervation is the obturator nerve.

(b) This is the m. gracilis which originates from the pelvic symphysis. It inserts onto the cranial border of the tibia and also makes a further contribution to the common calcanean tendon to insert onto the calcanean tuberosity. It is an adductor of the limb and a hip extensor and also aids in the extension of the tarsus. The innervation is from the obturator nerve.

(c) This is the m. sartorius which originates from the cranial portion of the ventral iliac spine and the region of the ventral spine. It has two apparent heads and bellies but inserts into the medial femoral fascia, and thus the patella, and the cranial border of the tibia. It is a flexor of the hip and protractor of the limb as well as producing some adduction. The innervation is from the femoral nerve.

(d) This is the femoral triangle which contains the femoral artery and vein along with the saphenous nerve trunk. The clinician is able to take the pulse rate here in the dog.

(e) This is the medial saphenous vein which contains blood flowing proximally from the distal limb.

206. (a) This is the m. vastus medialis which originates from the proximal femur and inserts onto the tibial tuberosity via the patellar ligament. It is an extensor of the stifle along with the other members of the quadriceps femoris group of muscles. Innervation is from the femoral nerve.

(b) These are two bellies of the m. semimembranosus which arise from the ischiatic tuberosity and insert onto the medial condyles of the femur and tibia. They are extensors of the hip joint and retractors of the limb. They can also flex the stifle to some extent because of the distal attachment.

ANSWERS

(c) This is the m. gastrocnemius which originates from the caudal border of the femur. As it courses over the caudal aspect of the femoral condyles the tendons of origin incorporate two small sesamoid bones, the fabellae, which articulate with the femoral surface. It inserts onto the calcanean tuberosity and is an extensor of the tarsus. Innervation is from the tibial nerve.

(d) Di is the patella, Dii is the patellar ligament and Diii is the tibial tuberosity. The m. quadriceps femoris inserts onto the patella and its tendon of insertion is continued distally from the patella as the patellar ligament to terminate upon the tibial tuberosity. The action of the muscle is transmitted through the patella to the tibia producing extension of the stifle.

(e) This is the common calcanean tendon (Achilles tendon) which has a major input from the m. gastrocnemius and the m. flexor digitorum superficialis. It also has a lesser input from the m. gracilis, m. semitendinosus and the m. biceps femoris. The multiple tendon is a result of this varied input.

207. (a) These bones are the tibia and fibula of a dog. Ai is the cranial face, Aii is the caudal face.

(b) Bi is the medial condyle, Bii is the lateral condyle. These are covered by the the menisci and approximated to the femoral condyles to form the femoro-tibial joints.

(c) Ci is the medial and lateral intercondylar tubercles demarcating Cii, the intercondylar eminence. Ciii is the caudal intercondylar area and Civ is the cranial intercondylar area. The cruciate ligaments arise from areas Ciii and Civ. The cranial and caudal tibiomeniscal ligaments are also found here as well as the transverse ligament between the menisci in the cranial area Civ.

(d) This is the tibial tuberosity onto which attaches the patellar ligament.

(e) Ei is the medial malleolus of the tibia. Eii is the lateral malleolus of the fibula. The medial and lateral collateral ligaments of tarsus attach to these.

208. (a) Ai is the stifle joint of a dog. Aii is the femoropatellar joint between the patella and trochlea of the femur. Aiii is the femorotibial joint between the femoral and tibial medial and lateral condyles with the medial and lateral meniscal cartilages interposed between the adjacent surfaces. Aiv is the proximal tibiofibular joint between the articular facets of the relevant bones.

(b) These are the lateral and medial fabellae which are found in the tendon of origin of the m. gastrocnemius. They form a protective layer for the tendons as they pass over the condylar areas of the femur.

(c) This is the sesamoid in the tendon of the m. popliteus.

(d) This is the muscular (extensor) groove in the lateral edge of the proximal tibia. This allows passage of the tendon of origin of the m. extensor digitorum longus.

(e) Ei is the tibial tuberosity. Eii is the distally running cranial border (tibial crest). The former arises from a separate centre for ossification and receives the tendon of insertion of the m. quadriceps femoris or patellar ligament. The latter receives tendons of insertion from the m. sartorius, m. gracilis and the m. semitendinosus.

209. (a) This is the os penis.

(b) These are fabellae which lie in the tendons of origin of the m. gastrocnemius; they protect these tendons as they play over the femoral condyles during movement.

(c) Ci is the joint space of the femorotibial joint, Cii is the lateral ridge, Ciii is the medial ridge of the trochlea.

(d) This is the patella. This glides proximally in the trochlea during extension of the stifle and distally during flexion.

(e) This is the joint space of the femorotibial joint. In life, this is not such a wide space as there are meniscal discs intercalated between the condyles of the femur and tibia as well as heavy deposits of fat. The cartilaginous discs do not image radiographically.

210. (a) These are the tibia and fibula.

(b) **Bi** is the intercondylar eminence, **Bii** is the medial intercondylar tubercle, **Biii** is the lateral intercondylar tubercle.

(c) **Ci** is the tibial tuberosity, **Cii** is the sulcus of the tibial tuberosity.

(d) This is the medial malleolus of the tibia.

(e) These bone are from a horse. The fibula is greatly reduced in its form distally and the body does not reach the distal tibial region. The distal epiphysis of the fibula becomes attached to the tibia to form the lateral malleolus. The presence of a sulcus on the tibial tuberosity is also indicative of a horse.

211. (a) This is the patella.

(b) These are the edges of the medial tubercle of the trochlea of the femur. The patella is found proximal to this in the extended stifle joint. This tubercle is extremely large indicating a horse.

(c) These are the articular surfaces of the femoral condyles. In the live animal they are in apposition with the meniscal cartilages which are attached to the proximal tibial surface.

(d) This is the tibial tuberosity onto which attaches the medial, intermediate and the lateral patellar ligaments.

(e) This is the supracondylar fossa. In the horse and ox it is a true depression for the origin of the superficial digital flexor muscle.

212. (a) This is the cranial aspect of the tarsus.

(b) **Bi** is the talus, **Bii** is the trochlea which articulates with the tibia.

(c) **Ci** is the calcaneus, **Cii** is the sustentaculum tali.

(d) This is the central tarsal bone. This articulates proximally with the talus, laterally with the fourth tarsal bone and distally with the first, second and third tarsal bones.

(e) The series is the medially placed first, second, third and the laterally placed fourth tarsal bones.

213. (a) **Ai** is the talocrural joint, **Aii** is the proximal intertarsal joint, **Aiii** is the distal intertarsal joint, **Aiv** is the tarsometatarsal joint. The greatest degree of movement is at the **Ai** where flexion and extension occur.

(b) This is the calcanean tuberosity of the calcaneus onto which inserts the common calcanean tendon. This is formed in the immature animal from a separate centre of ossification. There is also a centre for the body of the calcaneus which then fuses with that of the tuberosity.

(c) This is the lateral malleolus of the fibula to which attaches the lateral collateral of the tarsus. The ligament is divided into short and long portions. The former inserts onto the individual lateral tarsal bones while the latter runs to the fifth metatarsal bone.

(d) This is the dorsal sesamoid which is found on the dorsal surface of the metatarsophalangeal joint. This is intercalated in the tendon of the m. extensor digitorum longus.

(e) **Ei** is the ungual crest which is covered by the corium. **Eii** is the ungual process which is covered by the wall of the claw.

214. (a) These are the metatarsal bones, the second lies to the right, the fifth to the left. Long bones, developing from a centre of ossification for their body and centre for their distal extremity These fuse at the time of maturity.

(b) The mm. interossei are applied to the plantar surface of the metatarsal bones. Their tendons run distally to attach to the abaxial surfaces of the proximal sesamoids before continuing on towards the dorsal surface and merge with the tendons of the m. extensor digitorum longus.

(c) These are the proximal sesamoid bones which are held in place on the plantar surface by the collateral sesamoidean ligaments, the short distal sesamoidean ligaments, the cruciate distal sesamoidean ligaments and the intersesamoidean ligament.

(d) The tendons of the m. flexor digitorum superficialis and the m. flexor digitorum profundus are found in this space which is called the proximal scutum. They are held in position by the plantar annular ligaments

(e) These are the proximal, middle and distal phalanges which are all long bones by definition. The proximal and middle bones develop from a centre of ossification for the body and a separate centre for their proximal extremities, the distal bone develops from a single centre of ossification

215. (a) This is the talocrural joint.

(b) This is the talus.

(c) **Ci** is the calcaneus, **Cii** is the calcanean tuberosity.

(d) This is the fourth tarsal bone which lies laterally.

(e) This is the metatarsophalangeal joint. The paired proximal sesamoids, which are imaged superimposed upon the metatarsal bone, are lying immediately proximal to the joint.

216. (a) This is a metatarsal bone.

(b) This is the sagittal ridge which is located on the distal articular surface. This ridge lies in close apposition to a sagittal groove on the proximal articular surface of a proximal phalanx while, on its plantar surface, the two proximal sesamoids will be situated to each side of it.

(c) This is the metatarsal tuberosity onto which inserts the tendon of the m. tibialis cranialis.

(d) This is the vascular groove on the dorsal surface along which runs the dorsal metatarsal artery in life. The axial line also confirms the dual origin of this bone because in cross-section there is a division of the medullary cavity into two halves along this line.

(e) This shows evidence of a dual origin from Mt 3 and Mt 4 as there are two articular surfaces distally and the axial groove can be seen running along the dorsal surface. This indicates a ruminant species and the overall size suggests bovine.

217.(a) This is the body of the tibia.

(b) This is the edge of the distal epiphysis of the fibula which is separated from the tibia by a cartilaginous growth plate. This will eventually fuse with the distal tibia to form the lateral malleolus. This is only found in equidae as the distal fibula epiphysis is fused to the fibula body in most species. In ruminants it is a separate structure but it does not fuse with the tibia, remaining as a separate structure. This radiograph is of a young foal.

(c) This is the growth plate of the distal epiphysis of the tibia.

(d) This is the joint space and articular cartilage of the tarso-metatarsal joint.

(e) This is the talus which lies on the medial side.

218.(a) This is the tuber calcanei of the calcaneus.

(b) **Bi** is the talus, **Bii** is the ridge of the trochlea which contributes to the articulation with tibia.

(c) This is the central tarsal bone.

(d) This is the fourth tarsal bone.

(e) **Ei** is the second metatarsal (splint) bone. **Eii** is the fourth metatarsal (splint) bone. The calcaneus and the fourth tarsal bone lie on the lateral aspect of the joint, thus **Ei** is medial. This is the tarsus of a horse — the only species to have a fully formed third metatarsal bone associated with greatly reduced second and fourth metatarsal (splint) bones.

219.(a) This is the tendon of the m. extensor digitalis longus. This originates from the lateral epicondyle of the femur and inserts onto all three phalanges. This is from a horse.

(b) This is the m. interosseus or suspensory ligament. This arises from the proximal region of the third metatarsal bone. The ligament inserts onto the proximal sesamoids before travelling to the dorsal aspect to join the tendon of the long extensor of the digit.

(c) This is the straight sesamoidean ligament which runs between the proximal sesamoids and the complimentary cartilage of the middle phalanx.

(d) This is the tendon of the m. flexor digitalis profundus. This originates from the proximal tibia and fibula to insert onto the flexor process of the distal phalanx.

(e) **Ei** is the tendon of the m. flexor digitalis superficialis. This originates from the caudal aspect of the distal femur and inserts onto the proximal phalanx and the middle phalanx by its complimentary cartilage after dividing at **Eii** to allow passage of the deep flexor tendon.

220.(a) **Ai** is the tarsocruralis joint of the tarsus. The distal tibia, **Aii**, and the talus, **Aiii**, lie on either side of it.

(b) This is the tuber calcanei of the calcaneus.

(c) This is the tendon of the m. flexor digitalis superficialis which originates on the caudal aspect of the distal femur. It inserts at the level of the proximal interphalangeal joint onto the distal tubercles of the proximal phalanx and the complimentary cartilage of the middle phalanx.

(d) **Di** is the tendon of insertion of the m. gastrocnemius. **Dii** is the bursa which lies between the previous tendon and the tuber calcanei.

(e) This is the long plantar ligament which runs from the caudolateral surface of the calcaneus and inserts onto the third metatarsus. This ligament assists in supporting the tarsus during extension.

Index

Numbers refer to questions and answers

172